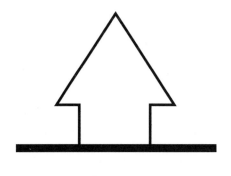

STRATEGIES FOR VALUE-BASED **PHYSICIAN COMPENSATION**

Medical Group Management Association

104 Inverness Terrace East

Englewood, CO 80112

877.275.6462

mgma.org

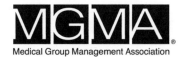

Library of Congress Cataloging-in-Publication Data
Milburn, Jeffrey B., author.
  Strategies for value-based physician compensation / by Jeffrey B. Milburn and Mary Mourar.
      p. ; cm.
  Includes bibliographical references and index.
  ISBN 978-1-56829-434-6
  I. Mourar, Mary, author. II. Medical Group Management Association, publisher. III. Title.
  [DNLM: 1. Evidence-Based Practice--economics. 2. Physician Incentive Plans--organization & administration. 3. Reimbursement, Incentive--trends. 4. Salaries and Fringe Benefits. W 80]
  HG9396
  331.2'16024610695--dc23
                        2013046376

Item #8652
ISBN: 978-1-56829-434-6

Printed in the United States of America

10 9 8 7 6 5 4 3 2 1

Contents

Acknowledgments... vii

Introduction ix

Chapter 1 ■ **Defining the Opportunity for a New Compensation Plan** 1

Historical Perspective 2
Is It Time for a New Compensation Plan?.......................... 5
Challenges Driving New Compensation Plans 7

Chapter 2 ■ **Managing the Compensation Plan Development Process**..... 17

Step 1: Define the Problem or Opportunity........................ 17
Step 2: Explore Information Needs................................ 30
Step 3: Collect Data... 31
Step 4: Interpret the Data 33

Chapter 3 ■ **Step 5: Size Up Alternative Compensation
Foundations** 43

Compensation Pool Determination 43
Selecting Compensation Models................................. 44

Chapter 4 ■ **New Reimbursement Systems and Value-Based
Compensation Incentives**.. 73

History of Payer Incentive Plans 74
New Reimbursement Models – What Are They? 75
Compensation Models and Value-Based Incentives 88

Chapter 5 ▪ **Special Issues in Physician Compensation** 107

Physicians' Career Stages. 108
Call Schedules and Compensation 113
Part-Time Physicians 115
Nonphysician Providers' Supervision and Revenue Distribution. 116
Large Group Practice Challenges. 118
Practice Leadership and Citizenship. 119
Ancillary Services and Designated Health Services Revenue 121
Compensation Pool for Special Issues 124

Chapter 6 ▪ **Legal and Regulatory Issues in Compensation Plan
Development** 125

Physician Employment Agreements 125
Legal Cautions. 129
Stark Law 131
Anti-Kickback Statute. 136
Accountable Care Organizations. 137

Chapter 7 ▪ **Plan Design, Approval, and Implementation** 143

Step 5 Continued: Size Up the Alternatives. 143
Step 6: Present the Information 147
Step 7: Determine the Outcome. 150
Step 8: Evaluate the Impact and Outcome 151
Start Over. 153

Chapter 8 ▪ **Integrated Physicians and Integrated Compensation:
Hospital and Health System Employed Physicians** 155

Goals for Integration. 155
Integration Models and Compensation Plans. 158
Compensation Plan Design Process in Integrated Systems. 160

Chapter 9 ▪ **Academic Faculty Compensation Formulas**. 171

History of Faculty Compensation 172
Faculty Compensation Plan Development 173
Academic Practice Case Studies 186

Chapter 10 ■ **Putting It All Together: Examples in Compensation Planning** 191

Simple Compensation Methodologies 191

More Complex Methodologies 195

ACO Examples – Incentives and Distribution of Shared Savings 206

Additional Integrated System Models 211

Appendix A ■ **Additional Resources** 215

Appendix B ■ **Understanding RVUs and the RBRVS System** 219

Appendix C ■ **Compensation per Work RVU Ratio Selection** 223

Bibliography 227

Index 235

About the Authors 249

Acknowledgments

We acknowledge the following whose contributions and advice are much appreciated in writing this book.

MGMA Health Care Consulting Group:

- Nick A. Fabrizio, PhD, FACMPE, FACHE;
- Kenneth T. Hertz, FACMPE; and
- Donna K. Knapp, MA, FACMPE.

MGMA-ACMPE Staff:

- Todd Evenson, MBA, director, MGMA-ACMPE Data Solutions;
- David N. Gans, MSHA, FACMPE, senior fellow, Industry Affairs;
- Laura Palmer, FACMPE, MGMA-ACMPE, senior industry analyst;
- Craig Wiberg, MBA, MLS, industry analyst; and
- MGMA-ACMPE Information Center staff: Marti Cox, Charlyn Treese, and Carol Welch.

We especially acknowledge the MGMA-ACMPE members who were willing to share their time, experiences, and knowledge on physician compensation and incentive systems. Their insights were invaluable in writing this book:

- David Cook, chief administrative officer, ProHealth Solutions, Waukesha, Wis.;
- Stephen W. Nuckolls, CEO, Coastal Carolina, New Bern, N.C.;
- Christine A. Schon, vice president, Community Group Practices, Dartmouth-Hitchcock, N.H.;
- David Taylor, vice president, Regional Services (Integrated Physicians Group), CoxHealth, Springfield, Mo.; and
- Shirley Zwinggi, administrator, and Steven Samuel, financial affairs manager, University of Texas Southwestern, Medical Center, Department of Surgery, Dallas, Texas.

Introduction

This book is intended to help medical practice and hospital executives develop and implement new physician compensation plans by:

- Understanding the various options in compensation models;
- Exploring the advantages and disadvantages for different models;
- Addressing practice-specific issues; and
- Introducing ideas to prepare for changing reimbursement.

Because designing physician compensation methodologies is a complicated issue and is critical to the recruitment and retention of physicians, it should be approached with diligent planning, physician participation, and careful implementation. For this reason, compensation planning is well suited for evidence-based management: a management decision-making process based on solid evidence and paralleling the idea of evidence-based medicine. Evidence-based management consists of defining a goal or objective, analyzing the current situation, and investigating information or data on examples, best practices, and trends to identify the best management plan or tactics to achieve the goal. Evidence to support decision making can come from qualitative data, published literature, and other sources.

The Medical Group Management Association (MGMA) has designed a tool to assist in incorporating evidence-based management in medical practices. Decision Pathways is a simple, repeatable process that moves you toward a crucial evidence-based management decision. It is available online at mgma.com and is defined as:

> *a systematic approach to addressing the critical elements that result in sound evidence-based management business decisions and lead to consistent, high-quality results for medical practice management teams.*

This book follows the eight decision steps in Decision Pathways in the process of compensation plan development, from initiation to implementation and evaluation. The eight steps are:

1. Define the problem or opportunity;

2. Explore information needs;

3. Collect data;

4. Interpret the data;

5. Size up the alternatives;

6. Present the information;

7. Determine the outcome; and

8. Evaluate the impact and outcome.

A historical perspective of physician compensation and the issues impacting compensation planning are described in chapter 1. Decision Pathway Steps 1 through 4 are discussed in chapter 2. Because of the complexity of Step 5, particularly in a time of changing reimbursement and incentives, this step is discussed in chapters 3, 4, and 5. Chapter 6 is dedicated to the complex legal issues related to physician compensation, including the Stark law. Chapter 7 finishes the Decision Pathway with the continuation of Step 5 as well as Steps 6, 7, and 8. The special issues of hospital-employed physicians and academic physicians are described in chapters 8 and 9. The final chapter includes many case studies of compensation plan development and implementation in a variety of settings to help the reader learn from peers who have completed the process. To assist readers interested in locating more detailed information, Appendix A lists additional resources, and the bibliography can be used to identify sources used in writing this book.

CHAPTER 1

Defining the Opportunity for a New Compensation Plan

Physician compensation plans are defined as the methodology for determining the amount of income that a physician will receive from the medical group practice or other entity. The compensation method can be via a guaranteed salary or a formula that is as simple or complex as the organization designs. It must be linked to the financial realities of the organization. In order to maintain the financial viability of the practice, compensation cannot be offered that is greater than the amount of funds available.

The three main objectives of compensation plans are:

1. Recruit and retain physicians by offering the opportunity for a fair and competitive compensation;

2. Ensure financial viability by balancing collections and practice expenses, including physician compensation; and

3. Align physician incentives and rewards with the healthcare organization's mission, vision, and values.

Compensation plans typically have additional objectives, such as increasing physician productivity, bringing in new patients, and addressing practice-specific issues. Each practice should determine its objectives prior to developing a compensation plan.

Since income can provide a sense of self-worth and esteem to individuals, compensation plans are also closely linked to physician behavior and self-esteem. Perceived inequities such as inadequate compensation or recognition of effort can affect physician satisfaction and retention. Compensation formulas can also be used as a means to provide incentives and rewards for specific behavior. David N. Gans, MGMA-ACMPE senior fellow, Industry Affairs, states

A physician compensation plan is a tool to encourage the right behaviors and discourage activities not consistent with the practice's goals. The right compensation and benefits package promotes productivity, improves quality, improves patient experience, and contributes to the organization's success. The wrong compensation and benefits package is disruptive and can fracture a medical group.[1]

With so much dependent on having the right compensation plan in place, plan development should proceed in a methodical, evidence-based manner ensuring physician input and buy-in to promote physician satisfaction and the organization's financial success. Because each practice is unique, the development process should not be shortcut by using a template or example from another practice. The plan must be developed by each practice to its characteristics and culture. A common saying among MGMA consultants and advisors is:

If you've seen one compensation plan, then you've seen one compensation plan. There are as many possible compensation plans as there are medical practices.

Historical Perspective

How to distribute practice revenue among physicians in a medical group practice has been an issue since the first two doctors decided to share an office. Because compensation is connected to many personal factors (pride in work, recognition for performance, lifestyle choices, etc.), it has never been an easy issue and has only become more complicated and contentious as society and healthcare have become more complicated.

For many years, physicians' take-home pay was what they collected from their patients for their services after they paid their staff, supplies, and office expenses. The method was jokingly called "keep what you treat" or "eat what you kill." In the early 1920s, physicians began joining together in medical groups seeking the advantages of sharing expenses, office staff, call coverage, and so on. Physicians in groups had to decide how they would share revenue after expenses. Since expenses were shared, would revenue be shared equally or would physicians track and keep their revenue after they paid their share of expenses? The question has continued to this day with new factors complicating the solution.

A multitude of studies show the connection between how people, including physicians, are paid and their behavior and job satisfaction. Henry Ford realized that if he paid employees more than anyone else, they would be happier longer while working on the mind-numbing automobile assembly lines. Employers soon learned that individuals can be encouraged to work faster, produce more, do an undesirable task, or improve customer satisfaction if their compensation or bonuses are based on or connected to any such factor.

Studies have also identified the complexity of developing incentives that encourage the desired behavior but do not increase undesirable behavior. Enough of the compensation must be based on performance to encourage the desired behavior. Incentives must be based on goals that are attainable but above the minimum expected performance to increase the performance to a higher level. Studies also show that individuals will learn how to "game" the system and use the incentives to improve their compensation but bring about undesired consequences.[2]

All of the above factors are true for physicians. Physicians generally respond to compensation plans by increasing the behavior that is rewarded with increased compensation, assuming compensation is a primary motivator. If the amount they are compensated is based on how much they charge or how much is collected from patients, they will charge more or perform more services. The U.S. healthcare system evolved from a structure where each patient paid the physician directly for rendered services to a system where insurers, covering patients' healthcare costs, pay physicians and hospitals for the services. However, both methods were based on a fee-for-service (FFS) method that meant physicians received more revenue, and therefore more compensation, the more services they performed. Analysis of MGMA Physician Compensation and Production Survey data show that physician compensation plans that are based on productivity levels result in higher collections than for physicians in practices that compensate via salary, equal share, or other nonproductivity-based methodology.[3]

The productivity-based compensation plan would seem to be the best method for medical practices, but it can result in undesirable consequences to the U.S. healthcare system. Increasing medical costs have required public payers (the federal and state governments through Medicare and Medicaid) and private payers (employers and commercial insurers) to look at alternatives other than the FFS reimbursement method. In the 1980s and 1990s, insurers shifted tactics and tried managed care. Managed care and health maintenance organizations restricted the physicians that patients could see to an approved network of physicians and paid them via capitation, a flat amount per assigned patient. Providers were now put at risk for services costing more than they received in the capitation rate. The push was then to reduce the amount of services, and medical practices had to rethink how physicians would be compensated under a model not rewarding production. The incentives shifted to cost-effectively managing the patient's total health services. A frequent result was providers and insurers denying patients services that they believed they had a right to or needed to maintain their health. The backlash resulted in a decline in capitation, so it is no longer common except in a few markets.

> **EXHIBIT 1.1 ■ Healthcare Expenditures as a Percentage of Gross Domestic Product, 2012**
>
> | | |
> |---|---|
> | United States | 17.0% |
> | France | 11.2% |
> | Netherlands | 11.1% |
> | Germany | 11.0% |
>
> Source: Data from OECD StatExtracts, Organisation for Economic Co-Operation and Development, Paris, France. http://stats.oecd.org/Index.aspx?DataSetCode=HEALTH_ECOR (accessed June 26, 2013).

With the decline of capitated managed care, health insurance costs continue to rise. In 2012, healthcare services totaled 17.0 percent of gross domestic product (Exhibit 1.1). Medicare and Medicaid was 21 percent of the federal budget in 2011.[4]

Changing Healthcare Reimbursement

With the realization that healthcare spending cannot continue to rise and increase as a percentage of total spending, healthcare and government leaders are looking at causes and alternatives for reducing the rate of growth in healthcare spending. Policy makers began asking why healthcare providers are paid on FFS regardless of the outcomes of the services. Ideas for reimbursing based on – or at least encouraging – quality, outcomes, and care coordination are being introduced. In the 2000s, the introduction of pay for performance or value-based reimbursement began. Hospitals and physicians are beginning to see incentives encouraging value and collaboration rather than volume. The 2010 Patient Protection and Affordable Care Act (PPACA) mandated changes in Medicare to transform healthcare payment and delivery systems. Risk-based reimbursement is returning in the form of bundled or capitated payments but including quality benchmarks this time. At the same time, hospitals and physicians increasingly see the benefits of uniting to form integrated health systems, and a greater percentage of physicians are now in practices owned or directly linked to hospitals and health systems.

Many efforts to restructure healthcare follow the principles of Triple Aim, a concept developed by the Institute for Healthcare Improvement (IHI) in 2008 by its then-president Don Berwick. The Triple Aims are:

1. Improve the health of a population;

2. Improve the patient experience of care; and

3. Reduce the per capita cost of healthcare.

The belief is that by combining all three factors rather than focusing on one over the others, the healthcare industry can gain efficiencies while improving the health of its citizens. Efficiency can be gained by combining per capita cost for a population and the experience of their care. Effectiveness is measured by population health and experience of care; comparing the effectiveness of alternative treatments and combining all of the factors results in the greatest gain.[5]

Are these new reimbursement methods here to stay? Will they become a major factor in reimbursement or stay as minor incentives? Will new methods be introduced? How much will the FFS model continue to be a component of reimbursement? Will hospital and physician integration last?

This book cannot answer questions about the future of the U.S. healthcare system, but its intent is to help practice administrators address the question: How should physicians in medical groups be compensated to meet the challenges of today and be prepared for tomorrow?

Is It Time for a New Compensation Plan?

Developing a new compensation model is frequently a painful process for physicians and administrators, and may seem like a process that is best avoided or delayed. However, the practice's physician compensation plan is a key factor in the success of the organization. Compensation affects physician satisfaction and hiring of new physicians. Compensation is also directly related to the long-term financial viability of the organization. It can be a key determinant of the productivity of each physician, and therefore the revenue, but it can also bankrupt a practice if compensation guarantees are too high. It is therefore imperative that the compensation model be fiscally responsible and in line with organization financial goals and culture, and provide a relative sense of equity among the groups' physicians.

Practice executives will know whether the compensation plan is not effective if any of the three objectives is not being addressed with the current system. Issues become evident when compensation threatens to exceed cash available for compensation, there are difficulties in recruiting new physicians, or physicians in the group are complaining about or even leaving the practice due to their compensation. Lack of alignment with organizational goals and objectives will be noticed when physicians' behavior is contrary to expectations or becomes a barrier in achieving goals. If the medical group has undergone a major change, the compensation formula should be reviewed to ensure it will still be effective and addresses internal and external challenges.

However, the need to change a compensation plan is not always obvious, and therefore the current plan should be reviewed periodically along with analysis of key performance indicators within the practice. How frequently the review occurs

> ### EXHIBIT 1.2 ■ Frequency of Plan Changes
>
> According to a HealthLeaders survey of health system and physician organization leaders, the frequency that organizations change their physician compensation plan is:
>   • Every 1–2 years: 41%
>   • Every 3–5 years: 38%
>   • 5 years or more: 21%
>
> Source: Data from Karen Minich-Pourshadi, "Physician Compensation Incentives Shifting," *HealthLeaders Media*, October 28, 2011, http://www.healthleadersmedia.com/content/MAG-272014/Physician-Compensation-Incentives-Shifting.html (accessed February 17, 2013).

depends on changes in the practice and marketplace and the severity or pace of the changes (Exhibit 1.2). Changes that may require reviewing and modifying or updating the plan include:

- More than two years since the last review of compensation plan incentives and the alignment with organizational goals;

- A significant change in the number of physicians or specialties within the organization;

- Industry and environmental modifications that require adjusting compensation to be competitive in marketplace (e.g., increase in competition for a particular specialty);

- Lack of desired behavior that is affecting organizational success, including poor participation in administrative activities, chart completion, and so on;

- An organizational or operational change that affects practice financials or physician behavior, including implementation of an electronic health record (EHR);

- Embarking on new strategic initiative, including new services, geographic expansion, or new payer relation; or

- Changes in the demographics such as age concentrations among the physicians with a large contingent approaching part-time retirement.

Other changes are more severe and the impact is great enough to require a new compensation plan. Examples of major changes include:

- Merger with another group practice or joining an integrated health system;

- Financial performance is declining;

- Patient satisfaction is poor resulting in decreasing volume;

- Major change in organizational strategic plan or goals, mission, or vision;

- Previous attempts to modify physician behavior have failed;

- Excessive complaints regarding current compensation plan or the plan is affecting or threatening physician retention;

- Payers are transitioning from FFS reimbursement or offering incentives to participate in value-based reimbursement; or

- The practice is planning to participate in new programs such as an accountable care organization (ACO) or medical home designation.

With these factors directly related to physician behavior and physician complaints, it is important to recognize whether or not the concern is with one physician or several. If one physician is showing inappropriate behavior, the issue should be dealt with directly by the practice executives and physician leadership rather than punishing all the groups' physicians by changing the compensation methodology to address one individual. If there is one physician complaining about the compensation plan, practice leadership must consider whether it is an individual objection or a sign of a deeper issue. The executives should consider whether or not the plan is equitable and if the underlying issues would remain in place if another physician is hired.

Interview the other physicians individually because they may consider the plan unfair but are afraid to speak up at group meetings. Physicians see how hard they are working compared to others in the practice and know the physician compensation numbers from surveys. They will know how their income compares with the market and how hard they are working compared to others. If there are concerns about inequity, they will need to be addressed. Inequity concerns may be due to physicians not fully understanding the current plan or using inappropriate realistic benchmarks for comparison. These issues should be explained during the meeting.

Challenges Driving New Compensation Plans

Changes in the medical practice and healthcare environment are pushing the need to update or rewrite compensation plans in medical groups. These changes spawn internal and external challenges that must be evaluated and addressed in compensation planning. Some of the challenges have been around for the history of medical group practices, but others are due to changes in the healthcare industry. The extent to which each practice is currently, or soon will be, impacted by these issues varies depending on the organization's history, culture, and marketplace. All should be considered during the process of updating or rewriting the compensation plan.

Internal Challenges

Rising costs have hit medical practices like many industries. The MGMA Cost Survey data show a 14.6 percent increase in total operating costs from 2007 to 2011.[6] Staff salaries and benefits continue to rise to match or beat inflation and employees' expectations. The largest increase in expenses over the same five-year period was in information technology expenses, which increased by 46 percent. This increase reflects the need for medical practices to invest in increasingly expensive practice management and EHR systems. Medical groups frequently deal with rising costs by encouraging physicians to raise their productivity or offer new services.

Larger practices have formed to unify efforts to negotiate with payers, compete in a changing marketplace, and support information technology purchases. The average MGMA physician-owned practice was 18.8 full-time equivalent physicians in 2010.[7] More physicians in a group can mean more complex issues and potential for dissatisfaction with the compensation structure, especially with a more diverse mix of specialties within the practice. Specialists brought in to provide a new service might complain that the other specialists don't understand or appreciate their specialty, its work load, and specific reimbursement issues. Primary care physicians (PCPs) in multispecialty practices may be jealous of the higher income of specialists while the specialists complain about subsidizing the PCPs. Under some compensation models, physicians practicing in poorer neighborhoods can suffer from lower collections and compensation than other practice members in wealthier neighborhoods because of payer differences. These are examples of the types of issues that will need to be considered in the compensation methodology.

Generational and gender issues can also complicate matters in writing the compensation model. Values and priorities can be different among generations. Younger physicians may not want to work as many hours or buy into medical practices. They may expect additional compensation for their share of call coverage. New-parent physicians or older physicians may request time off or part-time schedules while caring for a newborn child or family member. Certain physicians may prefer to spend more time with each patient than may be standard at a particular clinic or hospital setting, and thus their productivity levels will be impacted. Other physicians may resent or be jealous of these work and lifestyle choices. Experienced physicians in a practice may prefer individualized, productivity-focused compensation plans while younger physicians might prefer a guaranteed salary or equal share. These issues generate questions including how compensation for part-time physicians should be adjusted and how nonpartners will be compensated compared to partners.

New provider mix in medical practices is evolving as practices hire more nonphysician providers (NPPs). Nurse practitioners, physician assistants, and registered nurse anesthetists are incorporated in practices to support physicians and increase practice productivity and revenue. NPPs are also used to provide patient access when physician shortages make it more difficult to recruit physicians. Medical homes and increasing emphasis on coordinated care management encourage practices to hire care coordinators, nutritionists, patient educators, discharge managers, and so on. Physicians' roles may shift to include supervision of NPPs and team management. Recognition of these roles may have to be included in updated compensation methodology.

Practice culture is an important force in physician recruitment and retention and therefore in physician compensation foundations. A practice may be highly individualistic, more like "a group of practices" rather than a group practice. Compensation methodology in such a practice will be quite different than in team-based practices that may choose equal shares of revenue and expenses. Some practices may focus on providing care for the less fortunate or emphasize quality time with patients, and the compensation formula should support this culture rather than high productivity.

Practice leadership and administration are vital activities for the successful functioning of a medical practice. Physicians frequently serve roles such as managing partner, governing board member, medical director, and committee chair and participant. Some of these roles demand a fair amount of physicians' time and can reduce clinical time. If administrative time reduces clinical time and impacts compensation, physicians in productivity-based plans may be unwilling to serve in administrative roles. This issue leads to the question of whether or not physicians should receive compensation for this time and how that compensation will be determined.

External Challenges

Physicians and healthcare executives have less control over external issues but must learn to adapt to and thrive under the changes. Many of the challenges are due to healthcare reform, but others are the result of economic and industry changes. These factors must be considered in compensation plan designs since they affect recruitment, reimbursement, and compensation.

Reimbursement Changes Not Matching Cost Increases

Rising costs for medical practices have been greater than reimbursement rate increases. The Consumer Price Index increased 21.6 percent from 2002 to 2010, but overall changes in Medicare payments were less than 1 percent.[8] The MGMA Cost Survey data tracked an increase in medical practice expenses of almost 15 percent from 2007 to 2011.[9] For the same period, the Centers for Medicare & Medicaid Services (CMS) increased the resource-based relative value scale (RBRVS) conversion factor by only 4.9 percent.[10] Commercial insurance companies typically follow Medicare payment rates and have had similar minimal increases.

Medicare's sustainable growth rate (SGR) formula, which determines the Medicare fee schedule for each year, is flawed and requires congressional votes every year to avoid deep cuts in payments to physicians. The Medicare Payment Advisory Commission and healthcare stakeholders, including MGMA, have proposed various alternatives for fixing the system, but, at this writing, Congress hasn't approved any proposals.

It is increasingly difficult for medical groups to negotiate reimbursement rates since more than half of metropolitan areas in the United States now have one commercial insurer controlling 50 percent or more of the market. The payer that controls the market can dictate to medical practices what the contract will state, and groups have limited opportunity to negotiate unless they have a local size and/or specialty monopoly.

The increasing popularity of high-deductible health insurance plans and higher copayments has also changed reimbursement for medical group practices. Patients may delay physician visits and decline recommended but nonurgent services. Provisions in the PPACA requiring coverage of preventive health services may counter this trend. High-deductible plans also encourage patients to shop around and compare providers and prices before selecting where to have a service done. There is no longer a guarantee that a patient will stay with their physician's practice for additional services.

To make up the difference, medical practices look to increase productivity and revenues and lower operating costs. Physicians are encouraged to increase the number of visits or offer new services, and compensation methodology should consider how to promote such efforts.

Changing Demand for Physician Services

The aging population of the United States will continue to drive demand for PCPs and others that service the older population. Healthcare reform under the PPACA will aggravate the situation by increasing the number of insured by as much as 29 million, which could translate to an additional 25 million primary care visits.[11]

Several new reimbursement programs for Medicare and commercial payers aim to reduce healthcare costs by emphasizing primary care and intensive care management to reduce specialty services and hospital visits. The PPACA also requires coverage of many preventive health services with the goal of catching potential health issues before they become advanced conditions. These programs will further add to the demand for PCPs and increase compensation for primary care but may lower the need for specialists and the frequency of hospital services.

To recognize the importance of primary care services, the PPACA requires that state Medicaid payments to PCPs (family medicine, general internal medicine, and pediatric medicine) be increased to par with Medicare rates for 2013 and 2014 for evaluation and management services and immunizations. This Medicare/Medicaid primary care

EXHIBIT 1.3 ■ Change in Median Compensation 2008–2012

Primary care (family medicine, internal medicine, and pediatrics)	18.76%
All specialists	16.63%

Source: *MGMA Physician Compensation and Production Survey: 2013 Report Based on 2012 Data*, Englewood, CO: MGMA-ACMPE, 2013, p. 14.

payment parity rule has the potential of greatly increasing primary care revenue, especially with the expected increase in Medicaid enrollment under another provision of the PPACA.

Physician shortages have been predicted for several years. The Association of American Medical Colleges predicts the United States will see a shortage of 124,000 physicians by 2025, but the shortage could be greater with the expanded insurance coverage under the PPACA. The largest shortage, around 46,000, is expected to be for PCPs. The increased demand for PCPs may already be visible in changing compensation, as seen in Exhibit 1.3.

According to *MGMA Physician Placement Starting Salary Survey: 2013 Report Based on 2012 Data*, median first-year guaranteed compensation for PCPs rose modestly from $175,000 in 2011 to $180,000 in 2012, marking the fifth straight increase. Compensation decreased from $255,000 to $247,437 for first-year specialists.

To deal with physician shortages and changing demand, medical practices may have to increase what they offer to physicians of higher-demand specialties. This may be especially true in rural settings where physician recruitment has always been difficult. Integration of new physicians into a physician compensation plan at market salaries higher than existing group physicians may create issues unless other compensation levels are increased. Healthcare executives have also seen a shift from regional-based compensation comparisons to considering nationwide data in order to recruit physicians. Practices will need to adjust their specialty mix to include the services that will continue to be in high demand. Use of NPPs or physician incentives may be needed to maintain patient access and meet the increased demand for services. Alternative ways of thinking or providing services, including group or e-visits, may help meet the demand.

New Reimbursement Initiatives

With U.S. healthcare expenditures approaching 20 percent, there are increasing objections to the status quo and concern for the future, especially with the rising federal deficit and unsustainable growth of the Medicare and Medicaid system. The number of Medicare beneficiaries will double by 2020 to 80 million, and the number of Medicaid enrollees will increase under the PPACA. The CMS, health policy analysts, and congressional leaders are looking for alternatives to the current physician payment system, due to the flawed SGR formula, fragmented care, and paying by quantity of services rather than for quality.

Private insurers are also looking for alternatives to the FFS reimbursement methodology. One study identified the FFS system as the main cause for higher expenditures compared to other countries since "it contains incentives for increasing the volume and cost of services (whether appropriate or not), encourages duplication, discourages care coordination, and promotes inefficiency in the delivery of medical services."[12]

New initiatives are being implemented that seek to reduce healthcare expenditures but maintain and even improve quality of care. These initiatives take many forms but combine emphasis on quality, outcomes, and patient experience as well as cost efficiency.

The CMS initiated several changes to shift from paying for volume under the RBRVS FFS system to paying for quality and value. Other initiatives shift more risk to the providers or provide incentives to coordinate care among the hospital, physicians, and other providers. When the CMS leads with new initiatives, commercial payers often follow, affecting more of providers' reimbursement and revenue.

The new reimbursement systems involve four main models:

1. Value-based or pay-for-performance;

2. Medical homes and other care coordination initiatives;

3. Shared savings and ACOs; and

4. Shifting financial risk.

Value-Based Reimbursement. Also called pay-for-performance, value-based reimbursement is an "approach that bases rewards on improved quality, affordability of care and patient safety."[13] Pay-for-performance incentive programs use bonuses and/or withhold to reward providers for achieving quality and cost-of-care measures in conjunction with FFS reimbursement. The quality measures may be based on specialty society quality criteria or payer-developed criteria. Although value-based reimbursement has started slowly, it is expected to grow. For example, in 2012 UnitedHealth Group, the largest insurer in the nation, announced that value-based contracting will grow to include 50 to 70 percent of its network physicians by 2015.[14] Practices need to consider including incentives related to value-based factors in physician compensation plans.[15]

Examples of value-based reimbursement or pay-for-performance under Medicare include the Physician Quality Reporting System and the value-based reimbursement modifier. The latter offers differential payments under the Medicare Physician Fee Schedule to physicians or groups of physicians based on the quality of care furnished compared to the cost of care.

Medical Home and Care Coordination Initiatives. Care management or coordination is seen as an important factor in improving patient health and reducing costs by increasing patient contact and education, more intensively managing chronic conditions, and coordinating care between providers. Several initiatives are available from private and public payers to encourage care management or coordination through additional reimbursement to cover additional costs related to intensive patient management. Encouraging the medical home concept is one of the care management incentives.

Medical homes are characterized as "a physician practice and patient partnership that provides accessible, interactive, family focused, coordinated and comprehensive care."[16] Several associations and not-for-profit groups offer certification programs for practices that want to be recognized as medical homes or patient-centered medical homes.

Several private payers and state Medicaid programs recognize and reward medical homes through care coordination fees, increased payment for evaluation and management services, or quality and outcome bonuses.

Shared Savings and Accountable Care Organizations. Shared savings programs allow participants to keep any savings realized by the payer for specific services or the total cost of care per beneficiary or population. Some providers initiated efforts in gainsharing in the late 2000s with the goal of reducing costs through product and supply standardization, application of efficient treatment protocols, and improved care coordination. Most shared savings programs require physicians to unite efforts with hospitals in order to succeed, and therefore new alignment and cost control incentives need to be considered.

Accountable Care Organizations (ACOs), in one form or another, are used by CMS and several private payers as part of their shared savings programs to encourage providers to unite in a single entity to share accountability and rewards. The ACOs are expected to improve their patient population's health by coordinating inpatient and outpatient services and investing in infrastructure and redesigned care processes. The requirements to be an ACO vary by payer, but all are eligible to receive payments for shared savings after they meet quality performance and risk-adjusted utilization management standards. Most ACOs have developed clinically integrated networks to unite hospitals, physicians, and ancillary and other healthcare services.

Shifting Financial Risk. Financial risk-shifting initiatives have been initiated or reintroduced by public and private payers. Providers under such programs will be rewarded for cost-effectiveness while maintaining quality and experience of care or improving outcomes. Cost-effectiveness is essentially a combination of managing the costs and amount of care provided. Examples of risk-shifting reimbursement systems, in order of increasing risk, include the following:

- Case rate payments are single payments for the physician's services related to a specific diagnosis. They are frequently used for obstetrics services and include prepartum and delivery services and procedures.

- Bundled or case rate payments are single payments to cover the integrated care by inpatient or outpatient hospital services, physician services, and post–acute care services during an applicable episode of care (three days prior to admission and 30 days following discharge). The intent is to encourage cooperation among providers in efficiency and quality of care for specific diagnosis episodes of care. Since payment is less than the sum of previous payments, the entities must reduce costs while maintaining quality through standardization, managing length of stay, reducing readmissions, or other measures.

- Capitation, once in vogue in the 1980s and 1990s, is seeing a return. The intent is to replace the FFS, volume-based payment method with a flat payment usually calculated as per member per month. The fee is intended to cover all of the scope of services defined in the contract for a set population of enrollees. Global payments are a form of capitation intended to cover all patient care including hospital, ancillary, physician and other services, including pharmaceutical.

Although they are currently a small percentage of total healthcare reimbursement, these systems and models are expected to increase. Practices under more than one type of payment or reimbursement system may have to deal with conflicting incentives. Optimizing practice operations for one type of payment may not make sense for other payment methods. Incentives to increase volume of services will increase FFS reimbursement, but under bundled or global payments they will increase costs without increasing revenue and may actually result in losses if costs are beyond fixed payments. Emphasis on patient volume over patient experience or outcomes can impact reimbursement from value-based or shared savings programs. Emphasis on patient experience and outcomes for some programs can reduce FFS revenue from other payers. In developing compensation methodology, it is important to understand that optimizing practice and physician performance for one type of payment may lower profitability in other payment methods.

Integration and Alignment with Hospitals

The incentive to form ACOs has added to the trend of providers aligning with hospitals. However, integration has been an increasing factor in healthcare for many years. Physicians look to hospitals for help in the increased complexity and costs related to regulation compliance, information technology, and other investments. Integration also helps practices succeed in highly competitive marketplaces. In some cases, physicians may just want to get out of the problems of running a private practice by seeking hospital employment. Larger practices and integrated health systems are in a better position to negotiate contracts with commercial payers than smaller practices. Hospitals may seek practice ownership to participate in shared savings and other reimbursement programs that require clinical coordination and integration, although the main incentive for health systems is frequently market share and the additional revenue from physician services.

The percentage of physicians in hospital-based practices varies depending on which survey is used. Merritt Hawkins & Associates, the physician search firm, stated that requests for physician placements with hospitals represented 64 percent of all placements in 2012–2013 while placements for physician equity partnerships dropped to 3 percent. (Placements in group practices remained steady at 16 percent.)[17] Hospital ownership has increased from 35 percent of the total number of MGMA Physician Compensation and Production Survey participants in 2008 to 49 percent of the total participants in 2011. Todd Evenson, director of Data Solutions, MGMA-ACMPE, does acknowledge that the MGMA numbers are somewhat impacted because hospitals are more apt to report data because of legal requirements that the compensation they offer to physicians be based on fair market value.[18]

Compensation for physicians in hospital-based practices is different for several reasons. Hospitals must comply with specific regulatory requirements, and hospitals tend to look at their physician practices as "cost centers" and allocate overhead expenses in addition to administrative expenses. Also, hospitals generally don't distribute ancillary services income to physicians, whereas private practices have to determine how to split ancillary profit and losses. Other issues, including the potentially different incentives between the physician and hospital or health system and the complexity of decision making between system boards and physicians' practices, are frequent governance issues.

Most medical practices are currently facing some form of these challenges. Review of current and future issues needs to occur during the process of compensation plan development. Lack of consideration and inclusion will lead to a less effective compensation plan or one that doesn't align with the current group practice's financial and demographic situation and environmental influences.

End Notes

1. David N. Gans, senior fellow, Industry Affairs, MGMA-ACMPE, personal conversation with author, March 21, 2013.

2. Susan Reece Stowell, MBA, AVA, FACMPE, "Changing Incentives – Physician Compensation under Health Reform," ACMPE Fellow Paper (2011), http://www.mgma.com/workarea /downloadasset.aspx?id=1368310 (accessed January 18, 2013).

3. David N. Gans, MSHA, FACMPE, "What You Reward, You Get – And Lots of It," *MGMA Connexion*, 10, no.2 (2010): 17–18.

4. Devin Leonard, "Medicare and Medicaid Must Be Cut. Period," *Business Week* (November 8, 2012), http://www.businessweek.com/articles/2012-11-08/medi care-and-medicaid-must-be-cut-dot-period (accessed February 22, 2013).

5. Donald M. Berwick, Thomas W. Nolan, and John Whittington, "The Triple Aim: Care, Health, and Cost," IHI Innovation Series white paper (Cambridge, Mass.: Institute for Healthcare Improvement; 2012), http://content.healthaffairs.org/content/27/3/759.long (accessed February 28, 2013).

6. MGMA 2012 Cost Survey for Single Specialty and Multispecialty Practices, 2012 survey, MGMA Data Solutions Department.

7. MGMA, "State of Medical Practice – Integrated Delivery Systems," *MGMA Connexion* (January 2010), www.mgma.com/workarea/downloadasset.aspx?id=32156 (accessed April 27, 2013).

8. David N. Gans, "Data Mine: Keeping Up with Inflation," *MGMA Connexion* (January 2011), http://www.mgma.com/workarea/mgma_downloadasset.aspx?id=40536 (accessed February 12, 2013).

9. See note 6 above.

10. David N. Gans, MSHA, FACMPE, "With Increasing Costs, How Do Practices Maintain Their Bottom Line?" *MGMA Connexion* (January 2013), http://www.mgma.com/work area/mgma_downloadasset.aspx?id=1373084 (accessed February 20, 2013).

11. Elbert S. Huang and Kenneth Finegold, "Seven Million Americans Live in Areas Where Demand for Primary Care May Exceed Supply by More Than 10 Percent," *Health Affairs* 32 (2013): 614–621.

12. M.J. Laugesen and S.A. Glied, "Higher Fees Paid to U.S. Physicians Drive Higher Spending for Physician Services Compared to Other Countries," *Health Affairs* 30 (2011): 1647–1656.

13. Owen Dahl, "Objective Advice: Paying for Performance," *MGMA Connexion* (February 2011), http://mgma.com/WorkArea/mgma_downloadasset.aspx?id=40873 (accessed January 25, 2013).

14. Emily Berry, "United to Attach Performance Conditions to More Doctors' Pay by 2015," *amednews* (February 29, 2012), http://www.ama-assn.org/amednews/2012/02/27 /bisd0229.htm (accessed February 14, 2013).

15. See note 13 above.

16. Mary Mourar, *Experts Answer 95 New Practice Management Questions* (Englewood, CO: Medical Group Management Association: 2012), 256.

17. *2013 Review of Physician and Advanced Practitioner Recruiting Incentives* (Irving, TX: Merritt Hawkins, 2013), 4.

18. Todd Evenson, director, Data Solutions, MGMA-ACMPE, personal conversation with author, January 22, 2013.

CHAPTER 2

Managing the Compensation Plan Development Process

As mentioned in the introduction, this book will follow the eight decision steps in Decision Pathways to follow the process of compensation plan development, from initiation to implementation and evaluation. The eight steps are:

1. Define the problem or opportunity;

2. Explore information needs;

3. Collect data;

4. Interpret the data;

5. Size up the alternatives;

6. Present the information;

7. Determine the outcome; and

8. Evaluate the impact and outcome.

Step 1: Define the Problem or Opportunity

After the opportunity to develop a new or revised physician compensation plan is agreed on, the next step is to determine the process for approving and developing the compensation plan. Depending on the practice structure, as many physicians as practical should be involved in this step, but how decisions are made in the practice will impact the process for finalizing the goals and objectives.

Who Will Decide on the Plan?

Deciding who will develop the plan will be determined by the:

- Number of physicians in the practice;

- Type of practice: multispecialty, single specialty, and so on;

- Practice by-laws;

- Leadership structure; and

- Ownership of the practice or employer of the physicians.

Practice by-laws will state how decisions of this importance will be finalized. They should clearly state if compensation methodology can be changed by the governing board or requires a vote of the physicians. If a vote is required, can items be approved by a simple or super majority of the participants? Are a few physicians, such as the owners, allowed to veto any decision? If these issues are not clearly stated in the by-laws, they should be settled prior to the beginning of the process. It will only confuse matters if the question arises as the plan development is finishing.

If a super majority vote is required or vetoes are allowed, it will be more difficult to approve any changes, especially those that threaten their compensation. In these cases, the physicians in control should be actively involved in the plan development process or the group should consider modifying the by-laws prior to proceeding.

Physicians may be employed by a hospital or under an integrated system model, and approval authority for compensation changes may reside at a higher level. This will be addressed in chapter 8.

Compensation Plan Committee

Once the final decision-making process is determined, you can decide who will develop the plan. For small practices, the task may be assigned to a physician leader, the administrator, an administrator–physician team, or all of the physicians may work together. Because the final plan will have a major impact on the physicians personally, it may be better if administrators do not work alone but work in partnership with a physician or consultant. It is also important that the administrator be perceived as a neutral participant and not playing favorites during the development of the compensation plan.

Larger practices will want to designate a subset of the organization's physicians and personnel to devote time to the process since including all the physicians in the process could be too cumbersome and time-consuming for participants. This physician compensation committee will lead the assessment of the old plan and the investigation and development of a new plan. The committee should include physicians, administrative personnel, and an outside consultant if one is hired for the task. A financial officer or accountant is an important participant to include for the practice's business viewpoint and the ability to conduct data analyses on impact to practice financial performance and physician compensation. The practice's accountant or financial advisor can also serve as an outside objective voice and one with knowledge of the financial situation and impact of plan alternatives.

The committee should be separate from the governing board or other approval authority body to ensure different representation and a dedicated group separate from that body's responsibilities. It may be beneficial to have at least one member of the governing board or an approval authority representative participating so there is opportunity for their input. The representative should provide the approving group with progress reports in an effort to identify potential concerns early in the process. If the governing body is participating to some degree, the chances of approval will increase. Committee members should represent a diverse pool of physicians to bring different viewpoints and definitions of what is fair. Consider selecting a mix by specialty, age, number of years of experience or with the group, different departments or locations, and other characteristics. If some members are selected by the groups' physicians rather than its leadership, physician acceptance of a new plan may be easier to obtain.

Including an outside, objective voice in the committee should be considered because of the potential for discord in methodology design. Medical practice consultants bring wide experience to add to the discussion and an objective voice outside of the internal politics. Additional benefits of using practice consultants include:

1. Experience as facilitators in group negotiations to assist in reaching consensus;

2. Knowledge of alternatives in compensation foundations and methodology;

3. Assistance in identifying goals and objectives to align with organizational goals;

4. Ability to conduct modeling to analyze the impact of alternative plans;

5. Capacity to assume some responsibilities of the committee to free up time of other members; and

6. Ability to insulate the administrator from possible criticism.

Consultants can also absorb some of the unhappiness (or "take the heat") over alternative methodologies and their impact. A consultant can be freer to say what should be said that administrators frequently cannot say. See Exhibit 2.1.

The committee's charge should be defined and clear for the committee members so there is no misunderstanding on what is expected. The charge should support the development of the compensation plan's mission statement or guiding principles, as described later in this chapter. All of the group's physicians should be informed of the committee and its charge. An example is provided in Exhibit 2.2.

Committee Timeline and Communication Plan

The committee, in conjunction with the practice leadership, should set a timeline or expected implementation date. Providing a deadline will ensure that discussions don't continue endlessly, but the timeline should allow enough time to obtain input,

EXHIBIT 2.1 ■ Consultants' Potential Responsibilities in Compensation Planning

- Identify the current compensation plan's strengths and weaknesses;
- Benchmark current and proposed plans against market and peer group performance;
- Develop alternative structures;
- Match incentives to organizational goals;
- Develop alternative structures and measurement metrics;
- Lead formal presentations; and
- Facilitate decision making.

Source: MGMA Health Care Consulting Group, http://www.mgma.com/solutions/consulting.aspx?id=1060.

EXHIBIT 2.2 ■ Sample Physician Compensation Committee Charge

1. Determine goals and objectives of the compensation plan.
2. Develop a timeline and communication plan for accomplishing the task.
3. Investigate options for compensation methodology.
4. Identify relevant performance measures to align with organizational goals.
5. Consider an alternative methodology.
6. Test alternative(s) for market competitiveness, internal equity, and financial sustainability.
7. Develop a transition or implementation plan.
8. Present the recommended plan to the group and obtain consensus and approval.
9. Activate the implementation plan.
10. Conduct a post-implementation review.

explore theoretical options, and test options from a financial perspective. The compensation plan should be developed in a timely manner to reduce uncertainty and allow the practice to meet today's challenges. Six to nine months is usually a reasonable time frame.

It is important for the committee to develop a communication plan for informing practice leadership and physicians of the timeline and steps in the process. Nothing upsets people more than to have a committee or group "disappear into a black box" only to reappear with a plan of their own making. Physicians want to participate in the process and understand how the final product will be developed. The communication plan should include when and how the following information is shared:

1. Reasons for the new compensation methodology;
2. Decision pathway and steps;

3. Goals and objectives of the new plan;

4. Options for physician input;

5. Information gathered during the process;

6. Alternatives evaluated;

7. Financial calculations;

8. Final plan option(s) with examples of impact on individual compensation; and

9. A transition plan.

Communication should be provided at each step along the way using a variety of methods and presenters. It is not necessary to share all the information from the committee with everyone, but it is usually better to err on the side of too much information rather than too little. Early in the process, the practice leadership (board chair and/or executive) should present to the whole group the reasons a new methodology is needed. This communication should clearly state the internal and external challenges that require changing the compensation plan. It is important to gain acceptance of the need for change as early in the process as possible. The committee membership should be introduced along with the outside consultant if one is hired. This presentation should include graphs and charts to help physicians visualize the financial picture of the practice, recent trends, and projections: how much money is coming in, staff and operating expenses, and reimbursement trends or changes. These charts can be referred to later to demonstrate the limited pool of funds for compensation distribution and factors affecting that pool.

At appropriate steps during the process, the physicians should be informed via organization-wide or department meetings about the status of the process. Memos and e-mails should also be used to ensure that everyone receives the message. At some steps, individual physician interviews should be used, including when physician input is gathered at the beginning and when detailed information is shared regarding the final plan's impact on individual compensation. Individual meetings can be very productive in gaining input that might not be shared in group meetings.

Before implementing a plan, it is preferable to have individual physicians understand and buy into the overall plan concept and methodology before seeing their individual projected financial impact. Assuming a fixed amount of available compensation funds, any change to an existing plan will have a positive or negative impact on individual physicians. Physicians receiving an increase will rarely complain unless it isn't enough. Physicians receiving less may accept a small decline but will generally resist any material decline regardless of the reasons. In these cases, changes may have to be phased in to allow for individual adjustments.

Compensation Methodology Goals and Objectives

The first step in identifying a new compensation methodology is to determine the goals and objectives of the plan. The steps in this order are highly recommended for brand new or newly merged practices and for hospitals developing compensation formulas as they begin purchasing or forming physician practices. Identifying the plan goals and objectives early in the process will provide a unifying theme or target for the compensation committee to emphasize during the following steps in this process.

For already existing practices wishing to modify their current plan or develop a new plan, the compensation committee should consider delaying finalization of the plan goals and objectives until after data is gathered and interpreted (Steps 2 through 4). This will provide an opportunity to first identify current issues that need to be addressed after gathering physician input and analyzing benchmarking data. Committees in established practices should consider developing a mission statement or guiding principles at this point in time to guide them in the process and serve as a reminder why the process was undertaken. Plan goals and objectives will then be developed or finalized after collecting and interpreting information and determining what issues need to be addressed.

Aligning with the Organization's Mission and Vision

As previously stated, the plan must be aligned with the organization's mission and vision. The committee needs to answer:

1. What are our core values, mission, and vision?

2. What is our practice culture?

3. How do we measure success (patient satisfaction, payers' measures, productivity and revenue)?

4. What is the desired behavior to achieve success?

Mission and vision statements provide the framework for all operations and activities within an organization. They identify who you are, what you do and for whom, where you are going, and how you are going to get there. Mission statements define the organization's purpose and reasons for existence, and what the organization does and for whom. Vision statements provide the overall direction of the organization by stating how the organization defines success and where it wants to be in the future. The mission statement should form the frame of reference for the vision statement.[1] Ken Hertz, MGMA healthcare consultant, advises that "Vision is essential to make the rest of the pieces fall in place."

The group's culture should be the foundation of the mission and vision as well as the compensation methodology. Culture is defined as "a set of intangible characteristics displayed by the individuals in a group and the group as a whole. The current culture should be defined by those that live that culture."[2,3] It may not be easy to state the practice's culture, but it can be identified through the mission and vision statements and by interviewing physicians. The physician compact, if a practice has one, will help identify the culture by stating what a physician receives as a member of the group and what they are expected to contribute to the group. Examples of practice cultures are: team-oriented, competitive and individualistic, or service oriented. It is also possible to have multiple or competing cultures within a group. For example, a group with primary care physicians (team-oriented) and medical/surgical specialists (competitive and individualistic) can introduce an additional complexity into the compensation plan development process.

If the compensation plan does not align or, to some extent, address the organization's mission, vision, and culture, it will create conflicts and confusion over time. The plan could incentivize and reward behaviors that are contradictory to mission and culture. Physicians could be torn between complying with the practice's mission and earning the highest compensation. Resentment can build when some are rewarded for what others consider to be inappropriate behavior.

To fully understand the organization's mission and culture, the committee or consultant should review all of the practice's available, relevant documents including:

- Vision statement;
- Mission statement;
- List of values;
- Physician compact that defines what each physician receives as a member of the group and what he or she is expected to contribute to the group;
- Governing policies;
- Practice by-laws;
- Buy-in agreements and buy-out methodology;
- Strategic plans;
- Financial statements;
- Physician employment agreements;
- Current compensation plan; and
- Physician recruitment plans and policies.

In addition to these documents, the committee or consultant may ask the following questions:

- Does the payer mix and subsequent collections have material impact on different physicians and/or practice sites? Explain.

- What industry compensation surveys are currently utilized by the practice? How?

- How would you characterize your physician turnover rate?

- How has the current compensation methodology impacted your ability to recruit and retain physicians?

- Does the group have nonphysician providers, and if so, how should the plan address their revenue, expenses, and physician supervision time?

- How should ancillary services be addressed in the plan, if relevant to the practice?

- How is a compensation and benefit plan developed for new physicians?

- Are part-time physicians included in the practice? How is compensation addressed?

- What are the existing exceptions or "special deals" to the current plan?

- What are the primary administrative and physician concerns regarding the current compensation plan? What are its successes and failures?

- What other information should we be requesting for review that is important? Are there additional questions we should be asking?

Compensation Plan Objectives

It is important to develop a mission statement for the compensation plan that includes goals, objectives, ideal contents of the plan, and how success will be defined. The current or old plan can be measured against the new objectives as part of the initial assessment process. The mission statement can be developed by the practice leadership or compensation committee, or by all the physicians in a small practice. If the committee develops it, practice or organizational leadership should approve it. Several plan proposals have failed because they did not match the mission and goals of the overall organization or health system.

Examples of mission statements are given in Exhibit 2.3. Two of the mission statements include the concept of a "fair and equitable" compensation methodology. *Fairness* is a subjective term: what is fair to one physician will not necessarily be fair to another. Physicians typically include two types of equity in their personal "fairness" concept. Internal equity is in comparison to other physicians' productivity and compensation within the group. External equity is compensation and necessary productivity relative to physicians within the community and country. The assessment of the current plan should include identification of inequities. Several alternative methodologies should be reviewed and analyzed in terms of their equitability so that physicians will be reasonably rewarded relative to their work effort. Involving physicians in the development process will ease some of their concerns. Ken Hertz,

---

EXHIBIT 2.3 ▪ Examples of Mission Statements

*Create a fair and equitable physician compensation plan that advances the practice's mission and vision.**

~

Develop a non-arbitrary compensation system that is clear and understood by all and increases physicians' accountability for their performance and behavior.

~

Define "the approach that complements and fosters the group's missions, objectives, and corporate culture and is acceptable to and viewed as equitable by a large majority of the group's physicians."†

* Source: Decision Pathways, Medical Group Management Association, http://www.mgma
.com/ebm/DecisionPathways.aspx?id=1367361&step=1 (accessed February 16, 2013).
† Source: J.K. Levine, "Compensation Models and Issues for a Multispecialty Group Practice," *Journal of Ambulatory Care Management.*, 19(1996): 50–59.

EXHIBIT 2.4 ▪ Compensation Plan Guiding Principles

The following are examples of guiding principles for new compensation plans:
1. To value all missions within the practice and the community.
2. The perception of equitable distribution, which is essential to the plan.
3. Simplicity with well-understood incentives.
4. Easy to administer.
5. Comprehensive to address the internal and external challenges while keeping the simplicity principle in mind.
6. Flexible to incorporate expected and unexpected contingencies and marketplace changes. Administrative discretion may be needed for exceptional circumstances.
7. Linked to the organization's financial performance.

MGMA healthcare consultant, advises, "It may also be necessary for physicians to accept a plan that is 'equally unfair,' with no one or two physicians benefiting more than others." In addition, the early and ongoing involvement of physicians presents opportunities to educate them on what the reasonable methodologies are as well as market-driven compensation and production benchmarks to determine "fairness."

Along with or instead of a mission statement, the committee may want to develop a set of guiding principles (Exhibit 2.4) for the compensation plan. These principles will guide the development process and provide the framework for identifying the goals and objectives in alignment with the organizational mission and vision. We don't recommend that the compensation committee spend hours and multiple meetings attempting to wordsmith the perfect vision and mission statement with supporting goals and objectives. Develop the broad concepts, then begin work on the remaining steps.

Guiding principle No. 7 (in Exhibit 2.4) should always be on the minds of the committee and physicians. Everyone wants to take home as much income as possible; however, a practice will not survive if total physician compensation is greater than the net revenue after expenses. Even hospital or integrated systems have limits on how long or how many employed physicians they will subsidize.

After the committee has developed its mission statement or guiding principles and reviewed the mission, vision, and culture of the practice, it should start identifying goals and objectives of the plan. Goals are based on financial needs, what needs to change to achieve success as identified by the group, and what's not working in the current plan.

Examples of goals and objectives are shown in Exhibits 2.5 and 2.6, respectively.

EXHIBIT 2.5 ■ Goals of a Compensation Plan

- Construct a production-based compensation plan that encourages physicians to maintain reasonable productivity and rewards them according to their productivity.
- Provide the opportunity for physicians to earn competitive incomes – locally, regionally, and nationally.
- Avoid penalizing physicians when serving the group results in lower productivity.
- Provide a minimum guaranteed income or the opportunity to earn a minimum income.
- Set clear minimum-production standards and impose penalties for failing to meet standards.
- Provide financial incentives for behaviors that support the group's vision and strategic plans.

EXHIBIT 2.6 ■ Objectives of a Compensation Plan

- Create a "fair" or an "equally unfair" compensation method.
- Increase physician productivity.
- Encourage expense management with allocation of expenses that can be managed by physicians.
- Address special internal issues, including part-time physicians, administrative activities, and practice ownership issues.
- Integrate fiscal responsibility.
- Ensure regulatory compliance.
- Reward quality of care.
- Increase participation or citizenship with practice administration and other activities.
- Improve patient satisfaction.
- Recruit and retain new physicians.
- Improve physician satisfaction and retention.
- Promote team participation and service.
- Grow the practice in terms of the number of patients.
- Increase owner profits.
- Address changing trends in reimbursement.

Physician Input

Interviewing the physicians in the group will help the committee identify the objectives of the compensation plan. Obtaining physician input at this time will improve acceptance of the plan, help identify what a majority of the physicians want included in the new plan as well as the strengths and weakness of the current plan. Physicians should be asked several questions about the current system and what needs to be accomplished in the new methodology. Exhibit 2.7 is an example of a physician questionnaire. Encourage them to give the questions and answers considerable thought.

EXHIBIT 2.7 ■ Confidential Physician Compensation System Questionnaire

Please complete this questionnaire and return it to the consultant either during your confidential interview or as otherwise requested. All responses will remain strictly confidential.

Goals: Medical practice compensation systems promote different goals and behaviors. Please list the top three to five goals that, in your opinion, should be promoted in your compensation plan. Examples: productivity, patient satisfaction, quality, income sharing, expense control.

1. _____
2. _____
3. _____
4. _____
5. _____

Goal Achievement: Is the present plan meeting the above objectives? Why or why not?
_____
_____
_____

Current System Strengths: In your opinion, what is positive about the current system?
_____
_____
_____

Current System Weaknesses: What do you see as the primary weaknesses or problems with the current system?
_____
_____
_____

Current System Equity: In your opinion, is the current system "fair and equitable"? Yes or no, and why?
_____
_____
_____

Exhibit continued next page

EXHIBIT 2.7 ■ Confidential Physician Compensation System Questionnaire (continued)

Changes: What changes would you recommend for your system?

_____

_____

_____

Critical Issues: Are there any approaches or outcomes that would make a new or revised compensation plan unacceptable to you?

_____

_____

_____

Production Incentives: What percentage, if any, of the compensation formula should be based on individual physician productivity? _____%

Other Incentives: Should the compensation formula address other nonproductivity issues like patient satisfaction, clinical quality, expense control, group cooperation, and so forth? Why and to what degree? Should incentives be positive, negative, or both?

_____

_____

_____

Compensation Sharing: What percentage of available compensation should be shared equally? _____%. Why?

_____

_____

_____

Practice Expense Allocation: Should practice expenses be allocated to individuals through the compensation formula? How much? Why?

_____

_____

_____

Present Compensation Plan

Do you understand the present plan? _____

Can you explain the present plan to others? _____

Exhibit continued next page

EXHIBIT 2.7 ■ Confidential Physician Compensation System Questionnaire (continued)

On a scale of 1 (strongly disagree) to 5 (strongly agree), please respond to the following statements:

The current plan is fair and equitable to all.   _____

The current plan compensates me fairly for my work.   _____

The current plan is understandable.   _____

The current compensation plan needs to be revised.   _____

Other Issues: What other issues, if any, should be considered as part of this process? Call coverage? Part-time work? Retirement?

_____

_____

_____

_____

_____   _____

Your Name (please print)   Your Specialty

Physician Compensation Plan Questionnaire, © 2013 Jeffrey B. Milburn. Used with permission.

Meeting with physicians individually enables them to speak freely and honestly. In large physician meetings, a few individuals tend to dominate and others may be too hesitant to contribute. With small to medium practices, physicians can be interviewed face to face. In larger practices, questionnaires can be distributed to each physician and a representative sample interviewed in person. Every physician should participate in one form or another so there aren't complaints later that "I didn't have the chance to participate."

A good question to ask during the interview process is "Do you understand the current compensation plan?" and if the answer is yes, ask the physician to explain it. You may be surprised how many can't. It is a good practice to provide physicians with a summary written description of the current plan to include goals and general methodology along with a more detailed financial example for future reference.

During the interviews or when the questionnaires are distributed, have physicians identify the critical issues that must be addressed in the compensation formula. These deal breakers should be separated from items that physicians would like included but are not required. The committee should identify any unacceptable components or deal breakers that must be addressed versus other goals or objectives that are not considered "must haves." For example, some physicians may state that they will leave the practice if a minimum guaranteed salary is not included. In another practice, physicians will object if equal share distribution is included or if administrative time is not compensated for.

Ken Hertz, MGMA healthcare consultant, warns that when physicians are asked what is wrong with the current system, some are likely to reply, "I'm not getting paid enough." It is important to follow up on this statement and determine why the physician feels this way. It could be the physician is being paid adequately in relation to production and this can be demonstrated by sharing internal and external benchmark data. This may also be a good opportunity to explain again the realities of the practice's financial position. Graphs and charts should detail practice revenue and expenses, and what is left after paying expenses. The latter becomes the compensation pool – a finite amount of money available for distribution to the physicians. Explain that if this physician gets paid more, there will be less available for the other physicians. If revenue is declining or expenses are growing faster, then there is less left over. However, if revenue is increased or costs reduced, the amount available for physician compensation can increase.

After physician input is gathered, the committee can decide on the goals and objectives for determining the new compensation methodology. The committee should review the physician-identified deal breakers and how they align with leadership priorities and organizational goals. Objectives should be prioritized in terms of what must be included and what are secondary aims. This will help the committee prioritize items to include as components in compensation determination. Goals and acknowledged unacceptable components should be reported to the entire group for discussion and possible changes. Physicians will usually agree on the general objectives of the plan but may have different individual objectives, especially if they are at different career stages (young, experienced, retiring, etc.). There may also be debate about organizational and individual objectives and how to align them under the practice's mission.

Step 2: Explore Information Needs

With the goals and objectives identified and prioritized, it will be easier for the practice compensation committee to identify what information is needed to continue compensation plan development. Internal and external information should be gathered and analyzed to support decision making during the process. The following questions will help identify information needs:

- What issues have other practices faced when creating or revising their compensation plans?

- Are there examples of a compensation methodology that we can use and build on?

- How do our physicians' incomes and productivity compare to national and regional averages?

- What are the options and their advantages and disadvantages for measuring physician productivity?

- What is the relationship between productivity and compensation in similar practice settings?

- How can we influence cost containment and reducing expenses?

- How do we structure rewards and penalties to ensure behavior that supports our vision?

- What kinds of physician behaviors do other practices recognize and reward?

- What is the desired physician behavior to achieve our goals and objectives?

- How have other practices successfully managed compensation plan transitions?

- Is there a lack of participation in necessary practice administrative activities, and what are options to encourage that participation?

- What are options for rewarding nonclinical efforts such as marketing, educational presentations, and other activities? Are rewards necessary?

- Is there a demand for part-time schedules that the current compensation system doesn't address?

- Are any of our payers shifting away from paying solely based on fee-for-service? If so, what new payments or systems are they introducing?

- What Medicare innovative programs are we participating in?

- What measures are the Centers for Medicare & Medicaid Services (CMS) and commercial payers using to determine reimbursement under their new payments?

- Should we include and how do we structure rewards for meeting quality and excellence goals?

Step 3: Collect Data

With the large number of questions, information and data gathering can be divided among committee members or physicians. Tasks can be broken up by types and sources of data, including internal financial and clinical data as well as external industry resources. Administrative staff or consultants should be assigned some of these tasks since the amount of available information related to developing or fine tuning a compensation plan is significant. Typically, the nonphysician members of the committee have the time and resources to research and acquire information that can be packaged and provided to all the committee members so that everyone is exposed to the same information at the same time. The committee should be advised on what is available and agree to what they will use.

Many resources are available to review the various types of compensation plans, their strengths and weaknesses, and different ways to measure physician productivity. This book addresses many of the questions regarding compensation methodology alternatives for productivity and quality measures, along with expense allocation methods, but additional resources are available elsewhere that will provide case studies or dig deeper into some of the options. Additional resources (Appendix A) include articles, reports, networking with peers, hiring a consultant, and Internet searches. The MGMA Website includes many articles, webinars, member discussion groups, and the member directory for connecting with peers in similar practices.

For a comprehensive analysis of the current practice situation, a variety of data should be gathered, especially if payers are including quality and efficiency factors or introducing new payment mechanisms. New practices will not have current practice data to analyze but should still assess the practice environment population demographics of their community and the payer analysis for major payers in the community. Existing practices should include the following types of information to ensure that decisions are based on practice financial well-being: costs per patient and procedures, data gathering capabilities of the current information systems, and areas of concern that need to be addressed through the compensation system.

Financial data to gather and evaluate includes collection percentage, total medical revenue per physician, total operating cost per physician, total operating cost as a percentage of total medical revenue, cost per procedure or relative value unit (RVU), and total and work RVUs (wRVUs) for the practice and by physician. Additional financial information that should be reviewed includes aged accounts receivable, charge analysis, payment analysis, and adjustment reports. These reports should be broken out by physician, specialty, procedure code, payer type, and service location. In most situations, it is helpful to look at multiple years of data and identify and assess trends.

Patient care data should include number of referrals, inpatient admissions, length of stay, ancillary services, patient panel size, and patient satisfaction results. Request an appointment or encounter report broken out by physician, payer type, and service location, including next-available appointment and no-show analyses. Obtain claims data from payers to compare with the practice's electronic health record (EHR) data. Results of patient satisfaction surveys should be closely reviewed and compared to nationwide results. Do the results identify issues related to satisfaction, patient's experience, and access that could impact patient retention or patient referrals to the practice? Patient experience and access may also be factors in reimbursement incentives.

Payer analysis will include who are the key payers in terms of number of patients and reimbursement and what is their reimbursement rate. In primary care practices, include the percentage of patients assigned by payer and the percentage that can select their own physicians and services. In addition, the following questions should be answered related to payers offering quality incentives or new payment structures:

- What percentage of reimbursement is currently from quality incentives, bundled or capitation payments?

- What are the benefits of participating in new reimbursement incentives, and what is required to participate?

- What quality measures are being used, and what is the source of data to determine rewards or penalties?

- Are current practice information systems (practice management and EHR systems) capable of capturing, tracking, and reporting information needs, including process, outcomes, and structure measures?

- Has the practice been capturing this information or do additional steps need to be taken to capture and track needed information?

- Are physicians and medical staff completing EHR fields appropriately?

Step 4: Interpret the Data

The compensation committee or a subgroup of physicians should summarize the results gathered from the literature research, peers, and other sources. The literature and outside resource review can also be used to determine what key performance indicators are needed for comparing and designing compensation plans and projecting how variations would impact physician income. A subcommittee or the committee as a whole should evaluate practice data compared with external data in a benchmark analysis.

Critical Success Factors in Compensation Plans

The literature search and physician interviews should help the committee identify the important factors that will be key to the success of the newly developed compensation plan. The following are examples of critical success factors for a compensation plan:

- Aligned with organizational mission and values;

- Has internal and external equity in mind;

- Desired behaviors are incentivized;

- Doesn't offer compensation beyond available pool of funds;

- Trusted data systems are in place to calculate compensation and its components;

- Metrics are clearly defined, measurable, and within physicians' control;

- Unacceptable plan components and "must haves" or "deal breakers" are identified and addressed;

- Aligned with reimbursement sources and methodologies;

- Simple enough to be understood but complex enough to include necessary issues; and

- Not too complex to administer easily.

Every practice searches for the perfect compensation plan that is simple to explain, understand, and operationalize or administer. The reality is, in today's complex healthcare environment with multiple reimbursement methodologies and incentives, the ability to develop "simple" plans is diminishing but is still worth trying.

Benchmarking Practice and Physician Data

Benchmarking is defined as the "process of measuring and comparing performance internally and with external data to known standard."[4] Benchmarking enables administrators and the committee to evaluate, observe, and analyze current operations and financial status; determine areas of success and opportunities for improvement; and implement changes. Comparing and analyzing performance with a known standard offers an objective method of determining relative success or failure. It supports practice improvement and evidence-based management and decision making by reducing uncertainty. The goal of the process is to modify behavior and improve performance to achieve identified best practices.[5]

The benchmarking process relevant to compensation planning follows these steps:

1. Evaluate and identify the key indicators or what's important to track and change.

2. Observe how to track and record the data, especially out-of-office activity. If current systems aren't adequate, then new tools or spreadsheets are needed.

3. Locate sources of external data for comparison, including best practices and best-of-industry data. The more data sources, the better, including payer's and outside-the-industry data.

4. Determine metrics that measure the objective – Example: 75th percentile of nationwide physician compensation.

5. Analyze internal data compared to external benchmarks and determine the difference.

6. Adapt information learned into the context of your practice.

7. Determine action and options to incorporate in proposed compensation methodology.

8. Model possible changes.

9. Evaluate outcomes of changes to identify opportunities for continuous improvement.

Key indicators in physician compensation and production include total compensation, contributions to retirement, and productivity factors of collections, charges, total and wRVUs, and encounters. Practice financial data should also be benchmarked to assess the financial well-being of the practice compared with similar practices.

Benchmarking is used most successfully when key indicators to benchmark reflect the organization's and compensation plan's mission and vision, and the data and statistics are fully understood. It is important to compare apples to apples by understanding definitions of the external data and ensuring that internal data is configured to match the definition. For example, MGMA defines *physician total compensation* as "direct compensation reported on W2 or similar form minus any voluntary deductions such as 401(k), 403(b), Section 125, or Medical Savings Plan. Compensation should include salary, bonus and/or incentive payments, research stipends, and distribution of profits."[6] It is also important to consider whether contributions toward retirement are included in the compensation figures. For example, MGMA surveys consider employer and physician contributions toward retirement plans, including deferred compensation, 401(k), 403(b), or Keogh plans as a separate item, not included in compensation amounts. Review internal compensation data to see if a similar definition is used. Exhibit 2.8 offers additional rules to ensure success in benchmarking physician compensation and other group practice data.

Remember: The overall goal is to improve performance not reach a benchmark.

Healthcare Physician Compensation and Financial Surveys for Benchmarking

Several sources are available for gathering data on physician compensation and production. Very large organizations may choose to gather only internal figures to benchmark individual or department statistics. However, most practices will want to compare internal data with external survey sources. When deciding which survey is appropriate, look at the demographics of the survey respondents to see which most closely match your group (hospital or physician owned, small or very large). Look at more than one survey report, especially for specialties and subspecialties that have fewer practicing physicians. Sources for surveys include MGMA, other professional associations, specialty societies, regional medical societies, and consulting and recruiting firms. Exhibit 2.9 compares an MGMA survey with two physician compensation reports.

The reports typically break out data by multiple variables including region of the country, size or type of practice, and number of years of experience, which makes it

---

EXHIBIT 2.8 ■ Four Rules to Benchmark Practice Data

1. **Use the median instead of the mean.** The median is the midpoint of a set of data, while the mean is the average. Typically, it is more beneficial to use the median when benchmarking because the median is not affected by statistical outliers (extremely high or low numbers) that would affect the mean.

2. **Use survey tables that apply to your group.** Select data to compare practices and physicians that are similar to your group practice. Comparing data based on geographic location, practice type (multi- or single-specialty) and size, ownership, and physician characteristics will result in better analysis and meaning.

3. **Normalize your data.** When you have to compare your data to practices that are different types and sizes, you should normalize benchmarking data. Divide your data by varying units to assess multiple facets of your business. This will allow you to compare your data in several ways.

4. **Know that benchmarking is ongoing.** For full benefits, benchmarking your data with external data should be done on a regular basis to support continuous quality performance. For physician compensation and productivity, review comparative data on a monthly or quarterly basis.

Source: Madeline Hyden, "Data Benchmarking: Are You Following These Four Rules?" *MGMA InPractice Blog*, February 1, 2013. http://www.mgma.com/blog/data-benchmarking-are-you-following-these-four-rules/ (accessed February 12, 2013).

---

easier to look at data by different factors and their effect on the statistics. MGMA's online DataDive modules (www.mgma.com/datadive/) enable users to analyze survey data to a deeper level and crossing several variables. Exhibit 2.10 is an example of an MGMA DataDive table.

Practice financial data, including operating costs by type of expense, accounts receivable, and total revenue, can be benchmarked with the MGMA annual cost survey reports or the *MGMA Performance and Practices of Successful Medical Groups*. The latter report identifies better-performing groups to provide data on the "best in class" as a goal for improving your practice's performance.

Because of variation in survey responses from year to year, especially for specialties with limited responses, there are options for handling survey data for more accurate comparisons and to reduce the consequences of survey data fluctuations. The options to smooth benchmarking data include the following:

1. Use more than one survey and average their figures.

2. Use more than one table from a survey or multiple surveys and average the results.

3. Calculate the multiyear rolling average. For example, add three years' worth of data divided by 3 to determine an average: (Year 1 + 2 +3 = Sum) ÷ 3

4. Calculate the multiyear weighted average:
   (Current Year × 3 + Prior Year × 2 + Prior Year × 1) = Sum ÷ 6

EXHIBIT 2.9 ■ Benchmarking Resources Comparison, 2012 Reports

	MGMA*	AMGA†	Sullivan Cotter‡
Providers	62,000	55,800	~70,000
Practices	2,900	225	408
Single specialty	2,000	11	(Not available)
Multispecialty	900	214	(Not available)
Physician owned	800	85	Multispecialty practices: 47% Single specialty: 38%
Hospital owned	1,900	140	Multispecialty practices: 85% Single specialty: 12%

* Data from *MGMA Physician Compensation and Production Survey: 2012 Report Based on 2011 Data*, Medical Group Management Association.

† Data from American Medical Group Association, www.amga.org.

‡ Data from Sullivan Cotter and Associates, Inc., www.sullivancotter.com/.

EXHIBIT 2.10 ■ DataDive Table Example

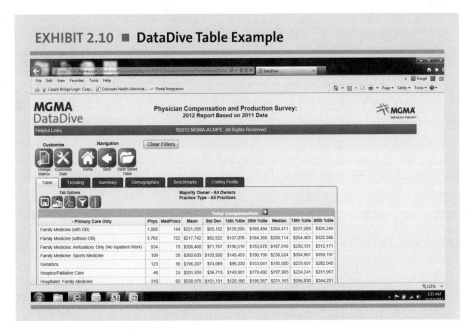

5. When using survey data to drive components of a compensation plan, consider setting floors and ceilings to accept in annual changes. For example, if a selected benchmark (median or 75th percentile wRVU conversion factor) changes more than 5 percent, limit the adjustment within the practice to ±5 percent. If the benchmark continues to change the next year, assume it's a trend and factor it in calculations subject to the annual floor ceiling change limitations until you catch up with the current survey metric.

Comparison Data Analysis

Develop charts to compare your physicians' compensation and productivity data including charges, collections, RVUs, and encounters. MGMA's Physician Compensation and Production DataDive product includes a benchmarking tool that generates comparison reports after you've entered your practice's and physician's data. Exhibit 2.11 is a sample ranking report showing one physician's data compared with the total practice and MGMA survey data. This sample report provides a one-page summary of each physician's relevant data highlighting when the rank is well below or above medians for other physicians. These comparison reports should be shared with physicians to clearly show their status compared to others within and outside the practice.

Along with comparing data from various measures, the ranking report lists ratios to demonstrate the relationship between the physician's compensation and productivity as measured by collections, charges, and wRVUs. By analyzing these ratios for all of a practice's physicians, it is possible to identify certain issues that need to be investigated further. If some physicians' compensation per wRVU ratios are much higher than others of the same specialty in the practice, then the current methodology may not be equitably distributing compensation based on work effort. Also if physicians' compensation per wRVU ratios are much higher compared to benchmarks than their compensation-to-collections ratio, then the physicians may be gaming the system by billing for services for which they won't get reimbursed but will add to their wRVU count. However, be very careful when using data to jump to a conclusion regarding "gaming the system." Although this is a possibility, it is also very possible the physician's location and payer mix contribute to a very low collection-to-wRVU ratio.

Sometimes you will see situations where your data doesn't make sense in relation to internal or external benchmarks. The amount of compensation earned or the time spent in nonclinical activities (administration, research, speaking, etc.) can impact total compensation and throw off compensation to clinical productivity benchmarks requiring adjustments to the data. For example, you may have a physician with median compensation and clinical productivity at the 25th percentile. Further investigation shows the physician has a half-time clinical practice and the remainder of the time is serving as a medical director. In this case, you will need to adjust the clinical production benchmark to half of the survey benchmark for a fair comparison.

It is useful to benchmark physicians' coding or procedural data to compare with MGMA, CMS, or other data to identify any outliers or inappropriate use of codes. For instance, many physicians will select the middle office visit Current Procedural Terminology® (CPT®)* codes (99213, for example) to limit the chance of being audited. Others may tend to select higher codes to boost their wRVUs. Accurate and appropriate

---

* CPT © 2014 American Medical Association. All rights reserved.

EXHIBIT 2.11 ■ Sample Ranking Report

Description for Doctor A*	Indicator†	Provider		Practice		MGMA	
		Value	Percentile Rank	Average	Variance	Median	Variance
Total Compensation		205,000.00	49th	202,500.00	1%	204,410.92	0%
Collections for Professional Charges (TC/NPP excluded)	+	515,000.00	75th	447,500.00	15%	392,747.00	31%
Compensation to Collections Ratio (TC/NPP excluded)	−	0.40	10th	0.46	−14%	0.56	−29%
Gross Charges (TC/NPP excluded)		670,000.00	52nd	585,000.00	15%	647,950.00	3%
Compensation to Gross Charges Ratio (TC/NPP excluded)	−	0.31	27th	0.35	−13%	0.35	−13%
Ambulatory Encounters (NPP excluded)	+	5,000.00	86th	4,250.00	18%	3,343.00	50%
Hospital Encounters (NPP excluded)		415.00	69th	307.50	35%	229.50	81%
Total RVUs (CMS RBRVS Method) (TC/NPP excluded)		12,000.00	74th	10,000.00	20%	9,703.15	24%
Compensation to Total RVUs Ratio (CMS RBRVS Method) (TC/ NPP excluded)	−	17.08	19th	21.04	−19%	22.57	−24%
Work RVUs (CMS RBRVS Method) (NPP excluded)	+	6,000.00	79th	5,000.00	20%	4,714.08	27%
Compensation to Physician Work RVUs Ratio (CMS RBRVS Method) (NPP excluded)	−	34.17	12th	42.08	−19%	43.63	−22%
Total Encounters (NPP excluded)	+	5,415.00	87th	4,557.50	19%	3,570.50	52%
Weeks Worked per Year		48.00	75th	48.00	0%	47.00	2%

Source: *MGMA Physician Compensation and Production Survey: 2012 Report Based on 2011 Data.* ©2012 MGMA-ACMPE. All Rights Reserved.

* NPP = nonphysician provider; RBRVS = resource-based relative value scale; TC = technical component.

† The Indicator column provides a quick reference to the doctor's ranking compared with the practice's and MGMA's medians. A "+" indicates that the doctor's values are at least 15% above the medians and a "−" means the values are lower than the medians.

coding will ensure proper reimbursement for services rendered and limit the concern about auditing.[7]

While conducting the benchmarking analysis, the committee should be asking questions such as:

- Which physicians are earning at or above the median compensation? Is their corresponding productivity at or above the median compensation?

- Does the data show lack of equitability in the compensation formula? Are physicians rewarded unevenly related to their work effort?

- Is the practice revenue above or below similar practices?

- How do physician encounters and RVUs compare among physicians in the practice and with external data?

Benchmarking Quality and Patient Satisfaction

Physician and practice comparisons should not stop at compensation and financial comparisons. An increasingly important factor in group practice success is quality of service and patient satisfaction or the whole patient experience. These are areas for possible improvement that can benefit from specific incentives, positive or negative, that are embedded in the compensation formula.

In this age of social media, potential customers are increasingly turning to their friends and online resources for help in selecting medical providers, similar to the selection process for choosing electricians or plumbers. Word of mouth has always been a key component for patient referrals, but social media enables a broader cast of the message and satisfaction. Websites have appeared that rank physicians based on patient satisfaction and quality factors. Health insurers, including Medicare, are providing enrollees with information that ranks physicians using formulas based on patient experience, quality, and cost factors. Medicare's Physician Compare, Anthem's Blue Precision, and UnitedHealthcare's UnitedHealth Premium are examples of payers' physician-ranking tools for enrollees.

Many group practices have been conducting patient satisfaction surveys for years. It is increasingly important for more practices to participate in satisfaction surveys that provide comparisons of survey results within the practice and with nationwide or regional data. This provides physicians an opportunity to see the results that potential patients can view. Medicare uses the Clinician and Group Consumer Assessment of Healthcare Providers and Systems (CG-CAHPS) survey. MGMA-ACMPE partnered with SullivanLuallin Group to build a tool that helps practices assess their current patient satisfaction levels and identify areas of improvement. The tool uses data from the CG-CAHPS survey to compare your practice's patient satisfaction data against national benchmarks.

Quality, outcomes, and cost-of-service data should also be reviewed and compared with available data. Internal data gathering may require information systems beyond EHR and practice management systems, including business or practice intelligence tools. Review data from the group's largest payers and request comparison reports. Appendix A includes a list of resources and contacts for quality and outcomes measures. Your practice may need to track the types of data previously not needed to achieve success under reimbursement systems that reward increased value (reduced costs). Physicians and administrators will need to track utilization including total costs to provide specific services or procedures and total patient services, including referrals, outside ancillary services, number of inpatient admissions, and length of stay.

Satisfaction, quality, and utilization comparison reports should help address the following questions:

- Is poor patient satisfaction reducing patient retention or referrals?

- Are poor patient satisfaction scores impacting practice revenue?

- Is there sufficient value-based reimbursement to include quality and value incentives?

- How do our quality, outcomes, and utilization scores compare to other physicians in the payers' reports?

- Are we losing marketplace share because of poorer quality or other ratings than other practices or physicians?

Finalize Compensation Plan Goals and Objectives

Compile the results of the physician input, benchmarking analysis, and literature review to identify what needs to be changed within the practice. This information should be used to finalize the goals and objectives for the compensation plan. Compensation committee members in already existing practices should review the information described earlier in this chapter (Step 1 in the "Compensation Methodology Goals and Objectives" section) to identify how to align plan goals and objectives with organizational mission, vision, and culture.

The goals will be dependent on what needs to be accomplished using compensation methodology to address the practice-specific issues identified during the previous steps. If practice revenue needs to be increased and/or expenses decreased, then these should be part of the compensation plan's goals. If the current compensation methodology is seen as inequitable and creating a sense of competition rather than camaraderie, then the goal should be to develop a more equitable formula. If the practice is struggling financially and current compensation levels are higher than benchmark data for the same level of collections, then the goals will emphasize bringing physician compensation in line with collections. Some goals may be dependent on the physician input that identified specific items which physicians have declared to be deal breakers or "must have" items and so must be included.

The final goals and objectives will drive the design of the compensation plan. For example, a goal to increase practice revenue should lead to compensation formulas that encourage and recognize physicians who increase their productivity. Incentives for bringing in additional revenue by offering new services or participating in promotional or marketing efforts could be added. If the current compensation methodology is seen as inequitable and creating a sense of competition rather than camaraderie, then the method could shift toward base salary or equal share. A goal of increasing participation in administrative functions will drive considerations on how to include compensation for participating in those functions. The identified need to improve ratings in satisfaction, quality, or utilization can be addressed by adding incentives or at-risk compensation based on physician improvements in these areas.

From the research, the committee will also have an idea of the general foundations for compensation methodology, the current and future payer reimbursement methods, and any other issues that need to be included. It is now ready for the next step to evaluate the alternative methods and decide how to include practice-specific issues and incentives to address changing reimbursement. Understanding the strengths and weaknesses of different compensation methodologies and incentives are discussed in the following chapters, which will assist in the decision and development process.

End Notes

1. Alan M. Zuckerman, *Healthcare Strategic Planning*, 2nd ed. ACHE Management Series (Chicago, IL: Health Administration Press, 2005), 46.

2. Todd M. Fowler, FACMPE, "From Recruiting to Provider Relations – A Mission-Critical Transformation," ACMPE Fellow Paper (October 2011).

3. Carol Westfall, "Group Culture: Medical Group Affiliation Levels and Effective Physician Recruitment," *NEJM CareerCenter Newsletter: Recruiting Physicians Today* (November-December 2003), www.nejmjobs.org/rpt/effective-physician-recruitment.aspx) (accessed February 1, 2013).

4. Mick Kasher and David Fein, "Benchmarking Physician Compensation and Production: Data Dive Compensation Module," MGMA webinar (January 28, 2009), https://mgmameetings.webex.com/mgmameetings/lsr.php?AT=pb&SP=EC&rID=5944532&rKey=f5ea63b538369984.

5. Ibid.

6. MGMA Physician Compensation and Production Survey, 2013 survey, MGMA Data Solutions Department.

7. Shawana Lynn Davis, FACMPE, "Using Benchmark Data to Evaluate Overall Practice Position," ACMPE Fellow Paper (2011). http://www.mgma.com/workarea/download asset.aspx?id=1368531 (accessed February 12, 2013).

CHAPTER 3

Step 5: Size Up Alternative Compensation Foundations

Step 5 in Decision Pathways is to *size up the alternatives*. In this and the following chapters the alternatives for compensation foundations will be discussed, including incentives and special issues in medical practices, along with legal and regulatory compliance in plan design. Narrowing the options in compensation plan design, the continuation of Step 5 is discussed in chapter 7.

There are as many physician compensation plans as there are medical practices, and it's impossible to say which formula is best for which type of practice. It is up to each practice to understand the basic alternatives or foundations, their strengths and weaknesses, and to decide which one aligns to the greatest degree with the practice's mission and culture. Within each compensation plan concept are options to customize the basic plan to incorporate the goals and objectives and to include practice-specific issues.

Compensation Pool Determination

No matter which compensation foundation is selected, the methodology must ensure that the group's total physician compensation is not greater than the amount of total revenue received by the practice minus all other expenses. Additional expenses include compensation for employed physicians and physician administrators who may not be under the owner compensation plan. The amount of money available for distribution in physician compensation should be determined first. This compensation pool is best calculated by estimating total revenue for a specific time period (one year or specific month) based on a rolling average of the previous several years' revenue and expenses. A rolling average allows for adjustments in month-to-month fluctuations. If there are positive or negative trends, factor them into your estimates. It may be necessary to exclude a particular month from the average if there was the sale of a large asset or a key producing physician was temporarily absent from the revenue stream. Revenue minus expenses becomes the practice's net operating profits available for physician compensation.

Also be aware that your accounting methodology – cash, accrual, or modified accrual – can impact your calculations. Principal payments on debt don't show up on the income statement but can certainly deplete available cash, and depreciation is shown as an expense on some financial statements but doesn't deplete cash. You basically need to know how much cash will generally be available for physician distribution. Looking at physician distributions over the last few years may be an adequate indicator for the future.

The group may choose to set aside a portion of net operating profits as a reserve fund or for capital purchases. However, the legal structure of practices will have different tax consequences. Physicians may also choose to distribute all taxable profits at each year end so the practice corporation is not taxed on the profits held in the corporation and then taxed again individually when distributed to owners. Tax issues are discussed in more detail in chapter 6.

An administrator can use the rolling averages of net operating profits to calculate the compensation pool, the amount of dollars available for physician compensation distribution. The pool can be determined on a monthly or annual basis. If calculated annually, actual revenue and expenses should be monitored monthly to ensure they are within expectations. A portion (usually 10 percent) of the compensation pool should be set aside to cover unforeseen situations. Distribution of the pool occurs with monthly or bimonthly payments to physicians based on the group's compensation methodology. At the end of the fiscal year, the withheld portion is distributed if revenue and expenses matched expectations. Remember, it is a lot easier (and safer) to withhold and distribute at the end of the year than to try and claw back money from the physicians in the event of a shortfall to cover expenses such as last-minute funding of retirement plans.

Selecting Compensation Models

Several basic compensation foundations or themes can be evaluated and selected. The foundations can be ordered or classified by administrative complexity, from simple to complex, as seen in Exhibit 3.1.

Simple Compensation Foundations: Salary and Equal Share

Straight or Guaranteed Salary

Straight salary can include a guaranteed salary for the year or a preset amount paid for each hour of work or shift. If the physician is not paid on a salaried basis and compensation is an hourly or per-shift amount, the physician may need to be compensated for any overtime work. The set amount is usually stated in an employment agreement or similar document when a physician first joins or begins working with the practice.

EXHIBIT 3.1 ■ Compensation Foundations – Administrative Complexity

Simple	Increasing Complexity	More Complex – Variable Driven	Very Complex
Straight salary	Salary or equal share with incentives	Productivity based	
Equal share	Equal and productivity sharing	Productivity plus expense allocation	Salary or equal share with value-based incentives
		Multiple components – hybrid	Productivity plus expense allocation plus value-based incentives

Advantages of straight salary for compensation include:

- Administrative simplicity – doesn't require calculations based on activity or determining collections;
- Can be market based using compensation surveys;
- Less stress on physician since compensation is a known amount and isn't at risk for other factors;
- Easy to budget;
- Not subject to frequent changes in demand or reimbursement;
- Supports the concept of a team effort and team-based culture;
- Decreased sense of competition encourages collaborative efforts;
- Doesn't encourage overutilization;
- Not impacted by participation in nonclinical activities; and
- Decreases individualistic attitude making it easier to implement changes.

Disadvantages of straight salary include:

- Not easily adjusted to changes in practice revenue;
- Doesn't provide incentives or rewards to encourage desired behavior, including increasing productivity;
- Not linked to ongoing financial situation of practice; and
- Not tied to use of resources or expenses.

Specific settings that straight or guaranteed salaries are most appropriate for:

- Hospitalists, radiologists, and physicians in emergency rooms or urgent care centers who can't control or have only minimal control of what happens during a shift, including patient demand or volume. These physicians are frequently paid by hour or shift rate or with an annual salary.

- New physicians who will have a period of being mentored followed by a period to build their share of a practice.

- Employees of a practice who choose not to buy into the practice or become shareholders.

- Specialties that have less demand but are recognized as a needed service within the community or organization. Health systems frequently use salary as a means of recruiting and retaining subspecialists for which there may not be enough demand to support a productivity-based compensation plan.

- Capitated or similar environment where reimbursement is not based on the volume of services provided.

- Team-oriented cultures with emphasis on care coordination and minimizing competition for patients.

- Established large medical groups with a strong culture and incentives to match performance expectations. Physicians are recruited that match the culture and are aware of the expectations regarding their behavior. These groups frequently attract physicians who are more adverse to risk than entrepreneurial smaller groups.

The **compensation pool** is calculated depending on the organization's status. Medical practices may incorporate salaries in the general compensation pool that funds all physicians' compensation or may include the dollars as an expense item that is deducted prior to determining the compensation fund. Health systems may incorporate salaries in department overhead expenses or as part of the general operating budget. In either case, expense allocation is not applied to the physicians' compensation determination.

Things to consider with straight salary are discussed in the following paragraphs.

The key to practice success with straight salary compensation is to ensure that the amount offered is within fair market value and physician expectations but not enough to bankrupt the practice. Physicians will also expect salaries to be in line with their seniority, experience, and previous compensation. It is important to conduct an accurate benchmark analysis to ensure that the offered compensation is within national or local market expectations and within the realities of the expected compensation pool. Too often, salaries have been set too high and thus affected practice and health system financial success.

Salaries for new physicians should be based on data from recruiting firms and surveys such as the annual *MGMA Physician Placement and Starting Salary Survey*. Depending on the marketplace and the specialty, starting physicians should be offered a salary for one to three years to build their practice before moving on to the compensation formula used for other physicians in the practice. If a new physician is taking over a retiring physician's practice with an established patient base, the new physician may be shifted to a productivity formula sooner than a new physician building a practice.

The major disadvantage of salary compensation is the lack of incentive to achieve and maintain productivity and thus an expected revenue stream for the practice. Organizations that offer a salary for new physicians or low-demand subspecialties may be willing to subsidize the salary, at least initially. Several options encourage productivity from physicians on salary. One option is a base salary plus incentive, discussed later in this chapter. A second option is to set minimal performance expectations to maintain employment. To provide an additional incentive to meet expectations, physicians can be offered extra compensation if they exceed productivity targets or they can be penalized if targets are not achieved. The latter option will place extra, unnecessary stress on starting physicians but can be used in other settings if realistic performance expectations are set.

For example, a physician must achieve a performance expectation at the MGMA 25th or 30th percentile of work relative value units (wRVUs) for the specialty to receive a full salary. Another method is to require the physician to work at least 90 percent of an FTE (full-time equivalent) schedule (measured by number of days or hours) or achieve 90 percent of an expected productivity measure (number of encounters, wRVUs, or collections) or else the salary is reduced by 10 percent or another amount. The performance expectations should be determined with the physician after careful considerations and analysis of benchmark data, the minimal expectations of the organization, and the physician's capabilities.[1] Patient demand is critical to support a productivity component. A physician on a productivity formula with no patients will quickly become discouraged. The group can also set expectations for timely submission of charge tickets, electronic health record (EHR) utilization, or citizenship activities to support practice administrative, marketing, or community efforts.

Mayo Clinic has used the salaried employment model since it began. The group believes that the major advantages include "physicians don't benefit individually from performing additional tests or unnecessary procedures" and it "encourages care coordination across the specialties and services." The latter is an important consideration in a large multispecialty practice.[2]

Equal Share Distribution

Another easy-to-administer compensation methodology is the equal distribution of the compensation pool, which is simple to calculate, as shown in Exhibit 3.2.

EXHIBIT 3.2 ■ Equal Share Methodology

This example is for a six-physician practice.

Practice net revenue	$3,000,000
Practice expenses	$1,800,000
Practice profit = compensation pool	$1,200,000
Number of physicians	6
Equal share of profits = compensation	$200,000

Advantages of the equal share methodology include:

- Administrative simplicity – doesn't require calculations based on individual activity or collections;
- Easily adjusted to changes in practice revenue and expenses providing stronger link to the practice's financial status;
- Directly linked to a team effort and supports a team-based culture;
- Lack of competition encourages collaborative efforts;
- Not impacted by participation in nonclinical activities; and
- Decreases the individualistic attitude making it easier to implement changes.

Disadvantages of the equal share methodology include:

- Doesn't provide individual incentives or rewards to encourage desired behavior;
- Less individual accountability since compensation is not directly tied to physician's individual effort or use of resources or expenses;
- More compensation is at risk than with a guaranteed salary;
- Possibility for resentment if belief develops that one physician (or more) is not "pulling his or her weight"; and
- Subject to changes in demand or reimbursement causing more month-to-month fluctuations than with salaries.

Specific settings that are appropriate for the equal profit sharing formula include:

- Single-specialty practices or specialties within a practice that are similar in reimbursement and resource demand;
- Practices that want to minimize internal competition for patients;

- Practices with physicians of compatible work ethic, productivity, and resource utilization; and

- Practice cultures where teamwork and team reward are a high priority.

Things to think about with equal share are discussed in the following paragraphs.

Individual physicians' direct expenses can be allocated or they can be expected to pay for malpractice insurance, continuing medical education, benefits, and so forth out of their compensation.

Including performance expectations as discussed under salary will help ensure that physicians maintain a minimal level of activity. Performance targets can be set for charges, collections, wRVUs, number of office visits, and/or number of clinical hours, and so on.

One pulmonary practice in Nevada has been successful under an equal share compensation method for several reasons:

- Physicians' schedules are equally distributed between the hospital, office, and the practice's sleep center;

- Because of the nature of pulmonary medicine, there is little control over which patients are seen in the office or hospital: whoever is on schedule sees the patients who present at that time for each location;

- Equal activity and schedules means equal share of expenses; and

- The practice is the only pulmonary practice in the community, so there isn't any need to incentivize physicians to increase patient numbers, which could also increase intrapractice competition for patients.[3]

Increasing Complexity: Adding Incentives

Salary or Equal Share Plus Incentive

Two major disadvantages of straight salary or equal share compensation are:

1. The lack of incentive to increase productivity or modify behavior; and

2. The weak link to personal accountability for costs.

The first factor can be lessened by including a portion of the available compensation based on an incentive. Receiving the incentive is contingent on achieving certain goals, following practice behavioral expectations, or contributing to the practice's financial success. Limiting the number and/or complexity of incentives can keep the

---

EXHIBIT 3.3 ■ Equal Share Plus Incentive Methodology

This example is for a six-physician practice.

Practice net revenue	$3,000,000
Practice expenses	$1,800,000
Practice profit	$1,200,000
Incentive pool −10%	$120,000
Net compensation pool	$1,080,000
Number of physicians	6
Equal share of profits = compensation	$180,000
Incentive pool distribution per physician	$10,000 to $30,000
Potential total compensation	$190,000 to $210,000

EXHIBIT 3.4 ■ Base Salary Plus Incentive Methodology

This example is for a second-year family practice physician.

Base salary	$150,000
20% Incentive opportunity	$30,000
Maximum potential total compensation	$180,000
Patient satisfaction >85%	$10,000
Productivity >60th percentile	$15,000
Good citizen	$5,000

---

plan relatively simple to manage. However, with more involved incentives and a higher percentage of compensation at risk, this option can evolve into a more complex plan to manage.

Exhibits 3.3 and 3.4 show examples of compensation formulas using different types of incentives.

The **compensation pool** is now two or more pools: one pool for the distribution of equal share or salary and the other to fund the incentive payments. The incentive pool can be funded by several sources:

1. Withholding of practice net revenue (as shown in Exhibit 3.4);

2. Separate funds from payers, health system, or other sources to fund quality improvement or support organizational goals and successes; or

3. Withholding a portion of an individual physician's compensation until specific goals or targets are achieved.

The third option is not recommended because it's inherently negative; physicians will see withholds as money they earned but won't receive until good behavior is achieved. Bonuses for agreed-upon behavior or extra effort are more appealing and don't carry a penalty.

Advantages of salary or equal share plus incentive include the advantages of salary and equal share distribution as described previously, as well as supporting a team environment and the security of a known compensation. Additional advantages include:

- Can be more closely linked to the practice's financial success;

- Increases a sense of personal accountability;

- Influences behavior to align with organizational goals and culture;

- Increased flexibility to adjust to changes in revenue, organizational goals, achievement of individual goals, and so on; and

- Motivates and rewards individual performance.

Disadvantages of salary or equal share plus incentive include:

- Base salary not easily adjusted to changes in actual practice revenue;

- Equal distribution can still generate resentment between physicians;

- Limited accountability for revenue and expenses;

- Difficulty in selecting appropriate percentage or amount of compensation for incentives that will motivate and what factors to include in payment calculation; and

- More complex to administer than straight salary or equal share compensation.

Specific situations that are appropriate for salary plus incentive include situations where guaranteed salary is preferred but the practice wants to encourage and reward desired behavior. This situation frequently includes new physicians and employed physicians.

Incentive Selection. As stated under the disadvantages for this methodology, the difficulty is in determining which measures will be incorporated in incentive plans and what percentage of compensation will either be at risk or high enough to motivate. For example, $5,000 to $10,000 will generally get the attention of a primary care physician but may not be enough to motivate a neurosurgeon. Sometimes nonmonetary incentives such as recognition, time off, or reduced call can be just as effective.

Incentives can be based on more than one factor, and there are several types of features that can be included. Two basic means for determining incentives are *objective* and *subjective*. Objective measures have the following characteristics to ensure they are trusted by physicians and administrators:

- Based on accurate and accepted data rather than opinions or observations;

- Within the practice's ability to record, track, and report;

- Known internal or external benchmarks for selection and comparison;

- Used to set realistic and achievable goals; and

- Within a physician's control.

The following are some examples of objective measures:

- Collections, wRVUs, or other productivity measures;

- Meeting attendance;

- Chart completion; and

- Quality or outcome measures.

Examples of subjective measures include communication and clinical skills and employee or peer relations. Since these are subjective, based on a medical director's or other individual's opinion, they may not receive as much weight as objective measures.

Patient satisfaction is both subjective and objective. It is subjective measurement when considering the part of the patient in completing the questionnaire or survey. However, the results or scores are fairly objective when compared to other physicians. If enough responses are received for it to be statistically valid, it can be considered an objective measure and is one of the more common quality incentive metrics used.

Productivity measures will be discussed later in this chapter. Quality, outcomes, satisfaction, and practice-specific activities will be discussed in more detail in chapters 4 and 5.

Percentage of Compensation. There is no magic number for determining what percentage of total compensation should be distributed via incentive or bonus. Each practice will have to determine for itself the right percentage depending on practice financial considerations, how much behavioral change is needed, physicians' control over the measure, and the source and amount of funds for the incentive pool, along with other factors. Reviewing the practice mission and goals along with the goals and objectives of the compensation plan will assist in determining priorities and how strong an influence on physician behavior is needed. The percentage should be high enough to affect physician behavior but not so high as to put too much at risk, increasing physician stress and resentment. It is better to start with a smaller percentage and increase it as needed over time rather than start too large and cause upheaval. A 10 to 20 percent incentive is often considered enough to get the physician's attention for productivity measures (collections or wRVUs), but incentive systems based on quality or satisfaction measures usually start with 5 to 10 percent.

The percentage of compensation based on incentive payments can also be increased over an employment period. New physicians may start out with only a small percentage of compensation based on incentive payments, but the percentage can increase after the first year.

Team and Individual Goals. Organizational or team goals should also be considered to enhance the team culture of a medical group. Team incentives will connect physicians with the success of the organization as a whole or by department or location. This also reflects that physicians are only one part of the operation along with many employees who also play key roles in achieving the goals and should receive a share of the incentive. Examples of team or organizational goals include patient satisfaction, achieving organizational financial goals, receipt of EHR meaningful use incentive, or achieving patient-centered medical home certification.

Equal and Productivity Sharing Combination

An equal sharing methodology can be modified to include additional components to increase the link between physician compensation with physician activities and success of the practice. The amount available for physician compensation can be divided into two pools, with one pool distributed in equal shares and the other based on different components. The additional components can include wRVUs, collections, revenue, and so forth; for example, 50 percent of the compensation pool distributed in equal shares and 50 percent based on a percentage of each physician's share of collections, total practice wRVUs, and so on.

Advantages of an equal and productivity sharing methodology include:

- Provides stronger link to practice financial status or physician activity;
- Offers opportunities to include incentives or rewards to encourage desired behavior;
- Supports a team-based culture;
- Lessens the potential for resentment that one physician (or more) does not work as hard as the others;
- Can encourage collaborative efforts;
- Minimizes the impact of participation in nonclinical activities; and
- Balances individualistic and team efforts making it easier to implement changes.

Disadvantages of an equal and productivity sharing methodology include:

- Less individual accountability since compensation is not directly tied to physician's individual effort or use of resources or expenses;

- More compensation is at risk than with a guaranteed salary or straight equal share; and

- Subject to changes in demand or reimbursement causing more month-to-month fluctuations than with salaries.

More Complex: Productivity Driven

As complexity increases, more variables and factors are included in compensation formulas. Compensation by a predetermined amount (salary or stipend) becomes a smaller portion of the total compensation or disappears altogether. Instead, compensation is based on variable factors that are more closely tied to physicians' behavior and use of resources. These plans can be more difficult to develop and administer but have enough advantages that they are a popular choice for practices.

Productivity-Based Compensation Methodologies

Physician productivity measures are the most frequently used variable in these plans. Productivity-based methodology has gained in popularity to encourage physicians to increase their productivity and therefore the practice revenue. This has been an effective means of combating the low rate of reimbursement increases compared with cost increases. Many practices have shifted to productivity-weighted plans to meet organization goals and improve the practice financial picture.

The basic formula for productivity-based compensation plans is:

$$\text{Physician Revenue} - \text{Expenses} = \text{Physician Compensation}$$

However, there are many details and factors to consider that add complexity to the basic formula. There are several methods for determining productivity-based compensation and several productivity measures to choose from. Also, should physician revenue be determined by charges, collections, RVUs, or another method? Should expenses be deducted from total practice revenue or calculated for each physician? Should compensation be based on each physician's revenue or as a percentage of total practice productivity?

The general concept of productivity-based methodology will be discussed first before describing the different productivity measures and their advantages and disadvantages.

Advantages of a productivity-based plan include:

- Increases physician accountability;

- Encourages and rewards a physician's effort to increase productivity and therefore revenue;

- Improves patient access because of incentives to see more patients and provide more services;

- Compensation is based on an individual physician's level of activity, decreasing complaints of others "not pulling their own weight."

Disadvantages of a productivity-based plan include:

- It is more complex to administer than salary or equal share;

- More of compensation is at risk to the physician;

- Physicians are rewarded for increased volume, potentially leading to overutilization;

- Potential exists for physicians to game the system through upcoding or encouraging patients to return more frequently than medically necessary;

- The plan increases competition among providers in the group, potentially decreasing care collaboration and adversely impacting the desire to hire additional physicians;

- Changes in revenue or reimbursement from one period to the next can increase the volatility of physician compensation;

- Nonclinical activities are not encouraged because of the potential impact on productivity and, therefore, compensation; and

- There is no direct link to quality, outcomes, or patient satisfaction.[4,5]

Specific Situations. Although the number of disadvantages is greater than advantages, productivity-based compensation plans are popular among medical practices because the fee-for-service (FFS) environment provides an incentive to boost productivity to increase revenue and therefore compensation. They are also being used by an increasing number of hospitals that employ physicians. A study of MGMA data by David N. Gans, MGMA-ACMPE vice president of Innovation and Research, about physician compensation and collections showed the link: "In each of the medical specialties examined, the median collections per physician were highest for the doctors who were paid by productivity-focused compensation systems. The increase in collections varied from 14 to 28 percent for physicians on productivity based plans versus salary based formulas."[6]

Productivity-based compensation can also be used in situations where physicians are reimbursed based on number of patient visits or patient panel size with the use of encounters or patients as a productivity measure. Practices that have less emphasis on team culture and more on individualism and personal accountability can do well under the methodology. The basic plan rewards physicians for their efficiency or high productivity but doesn't reward behavior that can support practice or team activities.

Keep in mind when looking at compensation plans with a productivity component that no matter what the physicians' productivity is, you still have to reconcile to the amount of cash available in the compensation pool. The pool is dependent on the amount and timing of cash available, less expenses. You can't, or shouldn't, pay out more than is available. Chapter 6 discusses regulations affecting total compensation distribution, including Stark law.

Productivity Measures. A physician's productivity is the most frequently used variable in this compensation methodology, and there are several productivity measures to choose from:

1. Charges;

2. Collections;

3. Work relative value units (wRVUs);

4. Patient encounters; and

5. Number of patients or patient panel size.

1. Charges. Professional gross charges is defined as "professional gross charges for individual physician and nonphysician provider productivity. The amount is based on the full fee schedule for the medical practice. It does not include the technical component, drug charges, supply charges, facility fees, or pharmaceutical charges."[7]

Since charges are based on the practice's own fee schedule, they reflect the actual work the physicians are doing compared to other physicians within the practice. Basing productivity on charges is payer-blind and doesn't penalize physicians whose patients are with undercompensating payers. However, since charges are always adjusted (usually lower) by payers, this measure doesn't reflect the actual revenue the physician contributes to the practice. Compensation based on charges may support income higher than the practice can afford, and physicians can game the formula by adding charges they know won't be reimbursed. It is also difficult to benchmark charges with external data since each practice sets its own fee schedule using a variety of methodologies. Charges don't take into account coding and billing issues or errors that result in denied or reduced claims. It is also difficult to increase charges without giving the physicians an automatic compensation increase that has little to do with productivity.

2. Collections. Collections or gross revenue is the actual dollars collected that can be attributed to a physician for all professional services, excluding the technical component of ancillary services and nonphysician providers (MGMA Physician Compensation and Production Survey). Collections reflect the adjustments made for payers' actual reimbursement and bad debt. For benchmarking purposes, MGMA determines collections as the total of FFS collections, allocated capitation payments, and payment for administration of immunizations and chemotherapy drugs. Another way to look at revenue from payers is to consider the contractual allowable on the Explanation of Benefits less their actual payment. The difference between the amount paid and the allowable is usually the amount paid by the patient. This represents the copayment that should have been collected at time of service and/or the balance to be billed to the patient. This amount isn't considered revenue until collected.

Compensation based on collections minus expenses may be the simplest and easiest to understand regarding productivity measures. Physicians understand: this is the money that I brought into the practice; subtract the expenses and I get what's left over. Collections reflect actual revenue in the practice and are better for external benchmarking since they are more closely linked to payers' reimbursement rates than charges. Actual compensation amounts are determined by specific collections brought in by the physicians or as a percentage of total collections. This productivity measure requires accurate accounting and billing to ensure that physicians are assigned the correct revenue for their services.

Because of the lengthy average days in accounts receivable due to the typical billing cycle, actual collections can be delayed anywhere from a few weeks to three months or more after a service is rendered. This can increase the volatility of physicians' compensation when based on collections. Administrators may have to educate physicians on why compensation fluctuates from month to month and the reason that a very busy month isn't reflected in a higher compensation that month. Also, collections are impacted by payers' reimbursement rates and a physician's mix of patients. The ability of practice management to negotiate good payer contracts is an important factor related to collections. To increase compensation, physicians may not accept patients from payers with lower rates, including Medicare and Medicaid enrollees. Since collections are also based on the effectiveness of the billing and collections department, physicians may pressure the billing department or believe they have less control over their actual compensation.

3. Work Relative Value Units (wRVUs). RVUs are nonmonetary, relative units of measure that indicate the value of healthcare services and relative difference in resources consumed when providing different procedures and services. RVUs assign relative values or weights to medical procedures primarily for the purpose of reimbursement for services performed. They are used as a standardized method of analyzing resources involved in the provision of services or procedures. The resource-based relative value scale (RBRVS) is the RVU system used by the Centers for Medicare & Medicaid Services

(CMS) in the Medicare Physician Fee Schedule. Commercial payers have also adopted the RBRVS or similar scales based on RVUs. See Appendix B for more details on RVUs and the RBRVS system.

The CMS RBRVS assigns a total RVU value for each Current Procedural Terminology® (CPT®) code. Total RVUs are then multiplied by a monetary conversion factor to determine the dollar amount paid to the provider for each service provided.

$$\text{Total RVU} \times \text{Conversion Factor} = \text{Payment}$$
$$1.5 \times \$40.00 = \$60.00$$

Medicare sets a fixed dollar conversion factor (CF) that is multiplied by a geographic adjuster to determine the payment allowable. Commercial payers will typically use the current Medicare CF or some multiple (higher or lower) of the Medicare CF to determine how much they will allow for the procedure. The payment will be the total allowable or some combination of the payer's payment and the patient's copayment and deductible.

Three components of RVUs are included in the calculation to determine total RVUs:

1. Provider wRVUs;

2. Practice expense RVUs; and

3. Malpractice expense RVUs.

Although the relative values are in theory based on actual expenses and work effort, they are actually to some degree arbitrarily determined by CMS with physician input. RVUs are still useful for benchmarking physician and practice activity and in determining relative expenses because of the standardization and widespread acceptance by payers. Either the total RVU or wRVU can be used for benchmarking physician productivity and determining compensation. Work RVUs are used much more commonly than total RVUs because wRVUs measure the time and effort of the provider.

The **advantages** of using RVUs versus other productivity measures include:

- High accountability for physicians' work effort – the more procedures and services, the more RVUs and the greater the compensation;

- Physicians can understand the link between RVUs and work effort to compensation;

- Payer blind – doesn't depend on payers' reimbursement per procedure so no disincentive for physicians to include Medicare or Medicaid patients;

- Effective measurement for external benchmarking because it is a widely accepted measurement in industry and industry surveys;

- Immune to the effectiveness of billing practices, contracting, and the billing and collections department; and

- Dependent on timely submission of accurate coding and documentation so it reinforces the need for physicians to accurately complete charges and records.

The **disadvantages** of using RVUs include:

- Encourages increasing volume and can lead to overutilization;

- Does not link with cost-efficiency unless cost allocation is also included;

- The RBRVS system emphasizes procedures over office visits – does not align with increasing emphasis on patient care management;

- Subject to CMS changes in RBRVS that will impact net revenue and physician compensation;

- No link to quality, outcomes, or patient satisfaction;

- Physicians can game the system by billing for services they know won't be reimbursed but will add to their RVU count; and

- Government and commercial payer selection of the CF will impact available cash for physician distribution.

Things to think about in adopting wRVUs as a productivity measure are discussed in the following paragraphs.

Practice administrators and physicians need to fully understand the RBRVS system in order to implement an effective compensation formula reflecting fairness within the practice and actual revenue. It is important to know the impact of periodic RVU adjustments. The annual Medicare Physician Fee Schedule should be reviewed for changes that will impact RVU values and reimbursement and how the changes will affect individual compensation relative to reimbursement, especially in multispecialty groups. The practice management information system and compensation formula should be modified to incorporate these changes. Additional suggestions to ensure accurate wRVU calculations in compensation formulas are included in Exhibit 3.5.

Examples of the RBRVS system adjustments that should be incorporated in the wRVU calculation are the use of and changes in modifiers and multiple procedure discounting. If modifiers and multiple procedure discounting aren't included in calculating the physician's wRVU compensation, then the actual compensation may reflect higher reimbursement than was actually received. Keep in mind, if a physician is credited with a greater share of the available compensation pool, it is coming out of the pockets of other physicians in the practice. Examples of modifiers that reduce reimbursement for a procedure include modifier 80 for surgical assistants, modifier 50 for bilateral procedures, modifier 51 for multiple surgical procedures, and

EXHIBIT 3.5 ■ Ensuring Accurate Work RVU Calculations in Compensation Formulas

1. Confirm the accuracy of RVU tracking in practice management and billing information systems.

   a. Some programs don't factor modifiers. An example is the "51" modifier for more than one procedure completed during one operation. Compensation should be adjusted to match payers' policies related to modifier reimbursement policies. Medicare's payment policies are frequently duplicated by other payers. Reimbursement can by adjusted from 0.1 to 1.5 depending on the modifier.

   b. Information systems are preloaded with the practice fee schedule and should be checked to ensure that the current year's schedule is in place. Examples of recent important changes are:

      • Medicare no longer paying for inpatient and outpatient consultation codes, and

      • An increase in wRVU values for office visits and the initial inpatient visit.

      Date of service needs to be matched with the correct year's fee schedule.

   c. Review how corrected and resubmitted claims are handled in the practice information system to ensure no duplication of wRVUs.

2. Conduct monthly audits to ensure the accuracy of RVU calculations at a procedure code level to identify any problems in a timely manner.

3. Know which services are included in bundled or global payments, especially for obstetrics and surgical procedures. Decide how these services will be included in the physician compensation calculation.

4. Hospital-employed physicians shouldn't include RVUs completed by other clinicians but billed under the physician's national provider identifier (NPI) number. Use appropriate modifiers instead.

5. Capture activities that have zero wRVU value, including procedures not listed in the RBRVS, as long as the physician is receiving reimbursement or other revenue for activity. Develop an internal RVU value based on similar procedures or relative work effort.

Source: Herd Midkiff and Elizabeth Cordaro (2012). "Developing Work RVUs for Production-Based Physician Compensation Programs." *hfm (Healthcare Financial Management)*, 66, no.6, 140–145.

modifier 59 for imaging reductions.[8] One solution is to insert into the group's RVU schedule or compensation formula a value for the wRVU with a modifier that is equal to the average percentage of reimbursement with the modifier. This works best in a single-specialty group with fairly equal work loads.

Don't feel limited by the given RVU values. Donna Knapp, MGMA Health Care Consulting Group, advises practices to consider modifying the wRVU values for compensation determination to reflect priorities in the practice. For example, a goal of the compensation plan is to increase the number of in-office services because physicians have reduced their in-practice time in order to increase the number of higher

EXHIBIT 3.6 ■ Individual wRVUs as a Percentage of Group wRVUs

	wRVUs	% of Group	Total Compensation
Doc 1	6,112	22%	$225,255.70
Doc 2	4,213	15%	$155,268.69
Doc 3	5,520	20%	$203,437.74
Doc 4	7,890	28%	$290,783.29
Doc 5	4,255	15%	$156,816.59
Total wRVUs	27,990	Total Compensation Pool	$1,031,562

EXHIBIT 3.7 ■ Individual wRVUs to Group wRVUs at a Single Value

	wRVUs	Compensation/wRVU Ratio	Total Compensation
Doc 1	6,112	$41.00	$250,592.00
Doc 2	4,213	$41.00	$172,733.00
Doc 3	5,520	$41.00	$226,320.00
Doc 4	7,890	$41.00	$323,490.00
Doc 5	4,255	$41.00	$174,455.00
Total wRVUs	27,990	Total Profit	$1,147,590

reimbursed hospital-based services. The RVU value of in-office services can be artificially increased to provide the incentive to increase time in the practice. Another example of a practice-initiated change is to increase the wRVU value for new patient visit codes as an incentive to bring in new patients and increase the physicians' patient panel. These practice-level changes will have no impact on payer reimbursement since billing and reimbursement is based on CPT codes. The pool of available reimbursement funds won't change, but the individual physician disbursement within the practice will change according to the compensation plan.

Compensation formula examples with wRVUs. Several methods can be used to determine the compensation based on wRVUs:

1. Determine each physician's percentage of the group's total wRVUs and determine their share of the compensation pool (see Exhibit 3.6). This method can also be done for other productivity measures such as charges, collections, and patient encounters.

2. Determine a compensation per wRVU ratio or value and multiply each physician's RVUs by the ratio (see Exhibit 3.7); or

3. Develop a tiered plan with compensation per wRVU value increasing at preset points of physician productivity levels (see Exhibit 3.8).

EXHIBIT 3.8 ■ Base Salary plus Tiered wRVU Values

	wRVUs	Compensation per wRVU Ratio	Base Compensation			
Established Group Standards	3,800	$41.00	$155,800			

Base wRVUs	Base Salary	3,801–4,500 wRVUs $38.00*	4,501–6,000 wRVUs $44.00*	6,001 or More wRVUs $50.00*	(plus Base)	Total Compensation
3,800	$155,800	—	—	—	$155,800	$155,800
4,800		$38,000	$13,200		$155,800	$207,000
6,000		$38,000	$66,000		$155,800	$259,800
7,200		$38,000	$66,000	$60,000	$155,800	$319,800

* Physicians earn additional production compensation above set RVU standard and have the opportunity to earn more per wRVU as they become more productive.

The key to options 2 and 3 is to determine an accurate compensation-to-wRVU ratio. This can be done by determining the total compensation pool and dividing by the number of wRVUs for the practice. The ratio can also be obtained by benchmark analysis using physician compensation and production surveys. The latter is the more frequently used method because it helps practice administrators determine market-based compensation figures that are specialty specific. The difficulty is in identifying the appropriate ratios.

In the compensation and production surveys, figures are typically presented in tables showing the median and various percentiles. The tendency in using benchmarking data is to select higher percentiles (75th or 90th percentiles) in compensation and production figures to provide goals and incentives for physicians to achieve high performance. For example, practices who want to compensate physicians at the 75th percentile, especially if their production is at the 75th percentile, will look at the compensation/wRVU at the 75th percentile. Using the data from the example in Exhibit 3.9, a practice may use $81.01 for the compensation/wRVU ratio. With compensation/wRVU ratios, this selection will backfire because the higher percentiles actually reflect highly compensated physicians compared to the amount of work performed. However, selecting lower percentiles favors the organization and requires more physician effort to reach higher compensation levels. Analysis of the calculations and data from an MGMA Physician Compensation and Production Survey show that it is better to use the median as a basis for determining the compensation/wRVU value. Appendix C includes a more detailed analysis showing why this is the case.

Tiered plans set a lower compensation per wRVU value for production at lower levels and increase the value at set points as the number of RVUs per physician increases. Physicians earn more per wRVU as they increase their productivity, as seen in

EXHIBIT 3.9 ■ Sample Compensation-to-wRVU Analysis

	10th percentile	25th percentile	Median	75th percentile	90th percentile
Reported compensation	$237,971	$345,647	$455,762	$616,400	$837,834
Reported wRVU	4,128	6,071	7,966	10,924	13,235
Reported compensation per wRVU	$38.60	$47.97	$59.00	$81.01	$104.95

Exhibit 3.8. Careful thought must be given to determining the compensation/wRVU value. Lower-tier values that are set too low may leave physicians feeling insulted, that their work is not adequately appreciated. On the other hand, a lower compensation/wRVU value for lower-tier wRVU values reflect that physicians have yet to cover the basic overhead or breakeven point. Once physicians have exceeded their breakeven point, their total RVUs are more valuable to the practice and more can be shared with the physicians. This is a strong motivator for physicians to achieve higher production levels. Values set too high can result in compensation higher than the organization can afford.

One of the disadvantages mentioned for basing compensation formulas solely on wRVUs is the opportunity for physicians to game the system by billing for services that add to their RVU count but for which they won't be reimbursed. Practice administrators should monitor the denials, nonpayments, and modifiers, and then reduce wRVUs accordingly. This will keep physicians from being paid more relative to actual collections.

Frank Cohen, consultant and expert on RVUs, offers that another option to counter this is by including collections as a factor in final compensation determination.[9] For example, 50 percent of compensation can be based on physicians' wRVUs and 50 percent on physicians' collections.[10]

4. Patient Encounters. *Encounters* are defined in the MGMA Physician Compensation and Production Survey as:

> *Documented face-to-face contact between a patient and a provider who exercises independent judgment in the provision of services to the individual. If a patient with the same diagnosis sees two different providers on the same day, it is one encounter. If a patient sees two different providers on the same day for two different diagnoses, then it is considered two encounters.*

There are two types of encounters: hospital and ambulatory. Ambulatory encounters can take place in any outpatient setting, including providers' offices, patient homes, urgent care centers, emergency rooms, and other outpatient facilities. Either total encounters or just ambulatory encounters can be used as a productivity measure in the compensation formula depending on the physician's setting and specialty. For example, many physicians in community health clinics or urgent care centers will not provide services in an inpatient setting, and the ambulatory encounters will equal their total encounters.

Advantages of encounters for a productivity measure include:

- External benchmarks are available; and
- It improves patient access with the incentive to see more patients.

Disadvantages include:

- They are not linked with actual revenue;
- Physicians can game the system in several ways; and
- They are not based on quality, outcomes, or satisfaction.

Specific situations where encounters are appropriate productivity measures include settings where reimbursement is based on a per-visit basis. For example, community health clinics or urgent care centers can encourage and reward physicians to see the maximum number of patients if there is a high patient demand. A study of one urban community health network switched compensation from straight salary to a set amount per encounter (from $22 and $30) and saw the average number of encounters increase from 11 to 60 percent, as well as the number of days at the clinics. They also included an additional amount per immunization, vaccination, and screening procedure to increase these preventive services.[11]

Physicians can game the system by telling patients to return for repeat visits when additional visits aren't necessary. An additional concern is the incentive to have more encounters per day or week by decreasing the time per visit, which can adversely impact the quality of care and patient satisfaction. This can be countered by benchmarking physician visits with internal and external data to identify abnormal activity and by monitoring patient satisfaction.

5. Number of Patients or Patient Panel Size. *Panel size* is defined in the MGMA Physician Compensation and Production Survey as:

> *The set of patients cared for by a physician as the number of individual unique patients that have been seen by any provider within the practice over the past 18 months.*

Specific settings where panel size is an effective measure of physician productivity include group practices that are trying to increase physicians' patient load and locations where reimbursement is based on panel size.

Capitation and global payments are dependent on the number of patients under a physician's or practice's care. *Capitation* is defined as:

> *Payment for the obligation to furnish all or part (e.g., physician professional services only within the scope of physician's specialty) of care for a given population of patients typically paid on a per beneficiary (member) per month basis (PMPM).*[12]

Since reimbursement is provided as a set amount to cover all healthcare services per member, the means of success include emphasizing cost-effective population health management. Although capitation was fairly widespread in managed care organizations in the 1980s and 1990s, backlash occurred because of the perceived effects of rationing healthcare and lack of emphasis on quality of care. The concept is being reintroduced by some payers in some markets, incorporating quality and outcome measures. Further discussion of this topic will continue in chapter 4.

Medical homes have also shifted focus from a per-procedure, volume-based payment to a per-patient, total care emphasis. As discussed later in chapter 4, reimbursement can be based on the number of patients, especially the number of patients with chronic diseases, although FFS may still be the main practice reimbursement methodology. You may end up administering two or more physician compensation methodologies.

Things to think about in using panel size for physician compensation includes whether or not reimbursement is dependent on cost and/or utilization management. If reimbursement is by PMPM, then utilization and costs above that amount will adversely impact the practice's finances. Compensation methodology should include factors or consequences to incentivize physicians to keep costs and utilization below expected amounts for their total patient panel. The capitation contract includes utilization outside of the physicians' control (i.e., specialty, hospital, and/or pharmaceutical services), so administrators should ensure that physicians have a fair amount of control in the patients' care. If patients are not directly assigned to a physician but are free to choose which provider(s) to go to, the physician will have little control over all the patients' services. Patient education must be a large factor in maintaining patient satisfaction to inform patients why some services are unnecessary and aren't being recommended.

Another factor is the severity of illness among patients within a physician's panel. This factor is independent of reimbursement methodology. Risk adjustment should be considered in determining a physician's panel size and ability to manage the population's health. For example, if one physician has 100 patients with diabetes out of 1,000 and another has only 50 in 1,000, then the workload demand can be quite different. CMS uses its Hierarchical Condition Category (HCC) model to calculate risk-adjusted reimbursement by diagnosis. The Risk Adjustment Factor (RAF) identifies an individual patient's status based on demographic characteristics and presence of chronic disease(s) or disease interactions. Private payers may have similar models or use the HCC-RAF model.

The practice should obtain the RAF scores for patients within the practice from CMS or other payers and use this data to determine the potential demand of effort of a physicians' panel. Coastal Carolina Health Care determines the average RAF score for its physicians' panels and increases compensation for those physicians with higher-than-average scores. This encourages physicians to continue to care for more patients with chronic conditions rather than to cherry-pick healthier patients.[13]

Productivity with Expense Allocation

The productivity examples listed previously utilized a compensation pool that was based on all net revenue (net operating profit) after total practice expenses. Practices sometimes choose to allocate at least some extraordinary expenses to physicians to increase the sense of responsibility toward operating costs and frequently allocate personal or individual business expenses within the practice. Some practices may identify expenses as a major problem and set up expense allocation as an incentive to reduce expenses. This doesn't always work if the physicians have little or no control over their expenses. It helps to look at the practice income statement or general ledger to see what expenses physicians actually have control over and can be motivated to manage.

To fully understand the expense allocations within a practice, we must understand the different types of expenses: fixed versus variable and direct versus indirect. Fixed expenses are those that are independent of the number of patients seen or procedures conducted. Examples include building and occupancy expenses (rent, utilities, information technology, etc.) Variable expenses increase as the number of patients or procedures increase. Medical and office supplies are the main examples of variable expenses. Staff salary and benefits are semi-fixed since they can be adjusted to meet practice volume but not quickly or easily.

Direct expenses are those that can be directly linked to an individual physician or department. Examples of direct expenses are physicians' retirement and other benefits, continuing medical education, malpractice insurance premiums, health and life insurance, professional license fees, and membership dues. Strict expense or cost accounting practices will also allocate many variable and staff expenses as direct expenses. Indirect expenses are the overhead expenses to support practice operations and include most of the fixed expenses and administrative staff expenses. These expenses cannot be directly assigned to individual physicians, but shares of these expenses could be allocated by share of one or more factors such as charges, collections, and patient visits.

The practice needs to link expense allocation, along with the rest of compensation methodology, with its culture and philosophy. Strongly team-oriented groups will include all expenses in one pool and cover the costs of physicians' expenses (up to a limit). More individualistic practices allocate as many expenses as possible.

Several options for allocating expenses are:

1. Equal share allocation;

2. Direct allocation;

3. Productivity-based allocation;

4. Mix of equal and direct allocation; and

5. RVU expense calculation.

Equal Share Allocation. With this option, all the expenses for the practice are shared equally among the physicians. Each share is then subtracted from the physicians' compensation, which was determined by the productivity measure. Physicians are made aware of expenses by seeing the effect of expenses on their compensation but are not personally accountable for their own expenses and utilization of resources. Equal share allocation works well in practices with team-oriented cultures and where specialties and production are fairly equal, and practice resource (space, staff, equipment) utilization is also fairly equal.

There are two possible methods for calculating the share. One is to combine all expenses to be allocated and divide by the number of physicians in the practice (shown in Exhibit 3.10). The second method (Exhibit 3.11) is to calculate the percentage of net revenue that is available after expenses. Each physician then receives as compensation that percentage of net revenue or collections attributed to their services. For example, if overhead expenses are 60 percent of net revenue, then 40 percent of revenue is available for the compensation pool. Each physician receives 40 percent of their net collections.

Direct Allocation. Strict cost accounting is required to track expenses per physician and subtract from their compensation. The accountability of costs and resource utilization is more directly linked to compensation under this method, but it is a more difficult and complex system to administer. This method works well when physicians want more staff, space, specific equipment, type of supply, or other individual expenses that are not shared by the group. Direct allocation also works well in practices with individualistic orientation and culture. Direct allocation may also occur in subgroups (per department or branch location) within an organization.

EXHIBIT 3.10 ■ Equal Share Expense Allocation

Practice net revenue/collections:	2,500,000
Practice total expenses:	1,250,000
Divided by number of physicians (5):	250,000

	Compensation Based on Productivity Measures	Expense Allocation	Total Compensation
Doc 1	$500,000	$250,000	$250,000
Doc 2	$422,000	$250,000	$172,000
Doc 3	$476,000	$250,000	$226,000
Doc 4	$573,000	$250,000	$323,000
Doc 5	$424,000	$250,000	$174,000

EXHIBIT 3.11 ■ Overhead Percentage Expense Allocation

Practice net revenue/collections:	$5,000,000
Total practice expenses:	$2,850,000
Compensation pool:	$2,150,000
Compensation pool as % of net revenue:	43%

	Collections per Physician	43% of Collections = Compensation
Doc 1	$755,000	$324,650
Doc 2	$1,245,000	$535,350
Doc 3	$630,000	$270,900
Doc 4	$1,370,000	$589,100
Doc 5	$1,000,000	$430,000
Total	$5,000,000	$2,150,000

Productivity-Based Allocation. Under the philosophy that "those who produce more use more resources," indirect expenses are distributed based on the percentage of physicians' individual productivity compared with the practice's total productivity. The formula (Exhibit 3.12) can be applied no matter which productivity measure is used (collections, wRVUs, or other factor), and the measure doesn't have to be the same as the compensation plan methodology. This option may be appropriate for practices with a wide range of productivity levels and cultures emphasizing individual effort. Direct expenses are usually allocated directly but can be included in the total expenses distributed by share of productivity. This method is similar to the second method in equal share allocation because the actual amount allocated depends on productivity, but in this option the percentage that is allocated varies by the percentage of a physician's productivity.

EXHIBIT 3.12 ■ Expense Allocation as Percentage of Group wRVUs

Total Profit:	$2,500,000			
Total Expenses:	$1,250,000			

	wRVUs	% of Group	Compensation Based on Productivity Measures	Ratio of Expenses Based on RVU %	Total Compensation
Doc 1	6,112	22%	$500,000	$275,000	$225,000
Doc 2	4,213	15%	$422,000	$187,500	$234,500
Doc 3	5,520	20%	$476,000	$250,000	$226,000
Doc 4	7,890	28%	$573,000	$350,000	$223,000
Doc 5	4,255	15%	$424,000	$187,500	$236,500
Total	27,990	100%	$2,395,000		$1,145,000

Mix of Equal and Direct Allocation. Medical practices with several departments or clinics may use a mix of equal and direct allocation. Costs related to shared overhead operations, including administration, human resources, and central billing office, are distributed equally among physicians or departments. Direct allocation to the department and its physicians is done for expenses such as rent, staff salaries and benefits, medical supplies, and equipment.

In order to balance team and individual efforts and rewards, a truly hybrid option is to share a percentage of operating expenses equally and the remainder by a percentage of the physicians' productivity compared to total practice productivity. This recognizes that all physicians share the benefits of some overhead expenses but that some expenses do increase as productivity increases. Which percentage to split the indirect expenses will depend on the type and culture of the practice. For example, a practice may choose to split 75 percent of the expenses equally and 25 percent based on production, or the split can be reversed or 50-50.

RVU Expense Calculation. This option is based on an expense per RVU calculation. Total operating expenses are divided by practice expense RVUs (peRVUs, not wRVUs) and then multiplied by the number of RVUs per physician (Exhibit 3.13). This method requires being able to separate peRVUs from total RVUs, since total RVUs contain physician work and malpractice components. The group must also be using the current RVU schedule and be aware of how changes in RVU weighting or assigned values in the RBRVS from one period to another will impact the cost allocation structure. For these reasons, this method for expense allocation is rarely used.[14]

Determining which of these expense allocation options is best for a practice will depend on the situation. Single-specialty practices with similar productivity and

EXHIBIT 3.13 ■ RVU Expense Allocation

Practice net revenue:	$2,500,000
Practice total operating expenses:	$800,000
Total professional expense RVUs:	16,000
Expense per peRVU:	$50

	wRVUs	Compensation per wRVU Ratio	Productivity Distribution	peRVUs	Expense/ peRVU	Physician's Allocated Expense	Total Compensation
Doc 1	6,112	$52.00	$317,824	3,500	$50.00	$175,000	$142,824
Doc 2	4,213	$52.00	$219,076	2,350	$50.00	$117,500	$101,576
Doc 3	5,520	$52.00	$287,040	3,250	$50.00	$162,500	$124,540
Doc 4	7,890	$52.00	$410,280	4,400	$50.00	$220,000	$190,280
Doc 5	4,255	$52.00	$221,260	2,400	$50.00	$120,000	$101,260

utilization demands may find that an equal share allocation is simple and appropriate. Direct allocation may work better in multispecialty practices with variable resource demands and revenue. Practices with limited ability or desire to track direct expenses can distribute based on a share of total productivity. Team-oriented practices might like the mix of equal share and allocation with a hybrid option.

Hybrid or Multiple-Component Systems

Compensation methodologies can include any mix of the previously discussed options. This next example is similar to the straight salary or equal share plus incentives option but with a greater percentage of the total compensation considered to be "at risk." For example, a practice may choose to base 60 percent of compensation on base or guaranteed salary and 40 percent on productivity. Another example is 50 percent based on equal share distribution of net revenue and 50 percent on productivity. The increased complexity of managing this methodology is due to the challenge of measuring and calculating the various factors. If a base salary is offered, it must be accurately determined or the compensation based on productivity can increase the total compensation beyond the limited compensation pool unless increased compensation is directly tied to the increased revenue produced under the plan.

An example of a hybrid system is one offering a base salary plus productivity compensation based on wRVU production. In the example seen in Exhibit 3.14, the base salary includes a performance expectation of 3,800 wRVUs. When that target is reached, physicians are eligible for additional compensation based on compensation per wRVU value for all productivity above the target.

Compensation formulas can even be split three ways to incorporate additional factors; for example, 50 percent distributed via base salary, 30 percent based on

EXHIBIT 3.14 ■ **Base Salary plus wRVU Production Paid at Single Rate**

	wRVUs	Compensation per wRVU Ratio	Base Compensation		
Established Group Standards	3,800	$41.00	$155,800		
MGMA Examples			Production Compensation	(plus Base)	Total Compensation
Median	4,500	$41.00	$28,700	$155,800	$184,500
75th percentile	6,000	$41.00	$90,200	$155,800	$246,000
90th percentile	7,200	$41.00	$139,400	$155,800	$295,200

Note: Physicians earn additional production compensation above set RVU standard.

collections, and 20 percent based on wRVUs.[15] A triple-split method can be appropriate where practices want to emphasize several factors or limit physicians from gaming one method to increase their income. Balancing compensation between collections and wRVUs, as recommended by Frank Cohen (described previously), counters the potential for physicians to inflate their RVU numbers. Triple-split formulas can also be successful in settings where physicians have a variety of responsibilities such as academic medical centers where faculty have clinical, teaching, and research responsibilities. (Academic faculty compensation is discussed further in chapter 10.)

Very Complex: Value-Based Incentives

The more complex compensation methodologies utilize multiple components in determining final compensation. Although they are more complex to develop and manage, they can be used to address a variety of goals and objectives and incorporate new incentives from new reimbursement systems. Combining productivity, expense allocations, quality, outcomes, and other factors within the compensation formula increases the connection between physicians and organizational goals and financial success. Examples of very complex compensation methodologies include:

■ Salary or equal share with pay-for-performance or value-based incentives; and

■ Productivity plus expense allocation plus value-based incentives.

Very complex methodologies need even more constant vigilance to ensure the accuracy of the variables and to determine whether or not total compensation is within the financial limits of the practice. With several variables, it is easier for the system to get out of alignment.

With the introduction of value-based or pay-for-performance reimbursement systems, medical practices are investigating basing a portion of physician compensation on the quality, outcomes, or patient satisfaction factors that payers are using for determining reimbursement. A portion of compensation can be dependent on physicians' scores or ratings on these factors while the remaining portion is determined by more traditional methods, including salary, equal share, or productivity. Because of the complexity of including quality, outcomes, and patient satisfaction incentives, this methodology is discussed in detail in chapter 4.

End Notes

1. William R. Greenfield, MD, "In Search of an Effective Physician Compensation Formula," *Family Practice Management*, 5, no.9 (1998): 50–57.

2. Robert L. Bratton, MD, "Salaried vs. Productivity-Based Physician Compensation: Advantages and Pitfalls," *Group Practice Journal*, 59, no.8 (2010): 38–43.

3. Donna Knapp, MA, FACMPE, MGMA Health Care Consulting Group, personal conversation with authors, April 10, 2013.

4. Alan Hill, "Show Me the Money: Developing the Right Compensation Structure for Your Practice," *MGMA Connexion* (August 2010). https://mgma.com/work area/mgma_downloadasset.aspx?id=34424 (accessed February 10, 2013).

5. Robert L. Bratton, MD, "Salaried vs. Productivity-Based Physician Compensation: Advantages and Pitfalls," *Group Practice Journal*, 59, no.8 (September 2010): 38–43.

6. David N. Gans, MSHA, FACMPE, "What You Reward, You Get – And Lots of It," *MGMA Connexion*, 10, no.2 (2010): 17–18.

7. "FAQs: Data Calculations and Glossary," MGMA Physician Compensation and Production Survey definitions, http://www.mgma.com/pm/default.aspx?id=9252 (accessed March 10, 2013).

8. Nancy M. Enos, "RVUs Are Your Biggest Chips in Physician-Employment Bargaining," *MGMA e-Source* (March 13, 2012), http://mgma.com/article.aspx ?id=1370192 (accessed February 12, 2013).

9. Frank Cohen, MPA, "Using Work RVUs to Compensate Docs: A Bomb-Proof Methodology" (presentation at MGMA Financial Management and Payer Contracting Conference, Phoenix, AZ, February 24–26, 2013).

10. Ibid.

11. Lorens A. Helmchen and Anthony T. Lo Sasso, "How Sensitive Is Physician Performance to Alternative Compensation Schedules? Evidence from a Large Network of Primary Care Clinics," *Health Economics*, 19 (2010): 1300–1317.

12. David N. Gans, "You Don't Know What You Don't Know: Information Needs for Future Payment Systems" (presentation at MGMA Financial Management and Payer Contracting Conference, Phoenix, AZ, February 25, 2013).

13. Stephen Nuckolls, CEO, Coastal Carolina Health Care, P.A., conversation with author, March 6, 2013.

14. David N. Gans, senior fellow, Industry Affairs, MGMA-ACMPE, personal conversation with author, March 21, 2013.

15. Bruce A. Johnson, JD, MPA, and Deborah Walker Keegan, *Physician Compensation Plans: State of the Art Strategies* (Englewood, CO: Medical Group Management Association, 2006), 235.

CHAPTER 4

New Reimbursement Systems and Value-Based Compensation Incentives

As mentioned in chapter 1, one of the external challenges facing medical group practices is the shifting reimbursement models from Medicare and other payers. The reimbursement systems are moving from reimbursing on a fee-for-service (FFS) basis to include incentives for quality, outcomes, improved patient experience, and reduced costs. The shift can be summarized as: Paying for value, not volume.

According to a Forbes Insights and Allscripts Healthcare Solutions survey of 204 hospital executives,

> *...73% agreed completely or somewhat that physicians needed to shift from volume to value immediately. Thirty-nine percent expected a quarter of total revenue to be linked to value-based purchasing within five years. Seventeen percent said it would comprise half of revenue.*[1]

In addition,

> *Physician compensation is expected to increasingly incorporate factors such as quality, outcomes and patient satisfaction. Incentive pay makes up 3% to 5% of the total compensation of employed physicians but is expected to be between 7% and 10% in the next few years, according to a survey of 424 health care organizations released Jan. 10, 2012, by Sullivan, Cotter and Associates.*[2]

Medical practices are also starting to include value-based factors in compensation formulas without being driven by external reimbursement. Incorporating these factors can instill the organizational emphasis on the patients' experience and health status that are frequently part of the mission, vision, and values of the practice or health system. Incorporating patient satisfaction, outcomes, and quality of care may be the most difficult of all the challenges for medical groups to incorporate in compensation plans. Although quality of care has always been a part of patient care, FFS reimbursement drove compensation models and physician behavior to emphasize volume, sometimes leading to overutilization, without factoring in quality. Value-based factors are also more difficult for administration to track and implement and for physicians to control compared to the number of procedures or collections.

Private payers have copied the Medicare models or developed their own systems. Several practices have negotiated with commercial payers showing the cost savings they've achieved with quality and outcomes management under Medicare. They were then able to negotiate additional reimbursement from new value-based contracts from commercial payers. State Medicaid programs have also introduced incentives, especially care management or coordination incentives.

Value-based reimbursement requires a shift of emphasis to ensuring that appropriate care is provided while volume is maintained. These reimbursement models require an organizational infrastructure to provide and track care in new ways but also a cultural shift to include emphasis on the new factors. Compensation plans can help with the cultural shift in providing the right incentives to adapt to the changing systems.

Although reimbursement under the new models is a small percentage of the total health system reimbursement, it is expected to increase and spread to affect more medical groups and health systems. Unfortunately, the shift is not occurring in a controlled manner. Different payers prefer different methods, placing groups and physicians in the awkward position of dealing with multiple and occasionally con-flicting incentives. Medical practices must rise to the challenge and opportunity of preparing for new payment systems while continuing to function under a largely FFS environment. Unfortunately, these new payment systems bring an unavoidable added layer of complexity that conflicts with the goal of keeping the plans as simple and understandable as possible. Compensation formulas must be flexible to prepare for new reimbursement incentives while maintaining the volume that is necessary for the financial viability of the practice.

In 2013, 11 percent of reimbursement to hospitals and physicians is value-oriented, according to the Catalyst for Payment Reform (CPR), an employer coalition. Of that 11 percent, 43 percent is bonus or incentive payments and 57 percent is at-risk pay-ments dependent on achieving quality and cost goals. Only 6 percent of physician payments is value oriented. CPR's goal is to have 20 percent of payments be value oriented by 2020.[3]

History of Payer Incentive Plans

Payer incentive and rating plans from the physician provider point of view have not been without problems. Lack of transparency regarding payer methodology has led to suspicions that the plans have been one sided in favor of the health plans, at least to some degree. One problem is the data utilized by payers was primarily developed from claims submitted by providers. This data could be incomplete if patients obtain services outside the payer network. If the incentive plan or a component of the incentive plan was specific to a single metric, then this would be easier to manage and audit. If the payer was using multiple metrics with different weights, it was difficult if not impossible for the provider to understand, much less audit the results. In some cases, the payer would utilize an inadequate sample size to develop their findings.

Quality rating systems could be equally problematic. Some payers would utilize a "proprietary system" to establish a physician or practice rating without disclosure of the metrics or weighted metrics utilized. Providers were concerned there might be an overemphasis on costs versus quality and that the plans were attempting to steer patients to low-cost providers regardless of quality. An extension of this would be when payers reduced the patient copayment for the more highly rated physicians or facilities.

Fortunately, the relationship between providers and payers has been improving over the years, and incentive plans and quality ratings are generally more transparent in their methodology. It is still recommended that providers perform their due diligence and totally understand the methodology utilized for incentives and ratings, and audit the payers' findings.

New Reimbursement Models — What Are They?

It is important to first understand the new reimbursement systems and their measurements and incentives. After describing these systems, we'll discuss methods of developing compensation incentives to align with the changing reimbursement methodologies. The four main models of new reimbursement systems are:

1. Value-based or pay-for-performance;
2. Medical homes and other care coordination initiatives;
3. Shared savings and accountable care organizations; and
4. Shifting financial risk.

The risk-shifting initiatives typically involve a payment mechanism that replaces FFS. The other three models maintain FFS as the basis and either modify the FFS payments or provide incentives in addition to the FFS payments. The differences create different incentives that groups must face to succeed under the different methods.

Value-Based Reimbursement

There are almost as many value-based payment or purchasing (VBP) models among payers as there are physician compensation models; however, the general definition is a payer or health system using reimbursement or bonus payments for the achievement of particular quality-related goals. These pay-for-performance (P4P) systems have several things in common:

- Based on metrics or measures;
- Not based on volume of services (although FFS may still underlie the whole reimbursement system);
- Frequently include efficiency or cost savings goals; and
- Include additional payment for achieving set goals or measures.

Value or performance-based contracting maintains existing FFS or capitation payment methods but ties payment increases or other incentives to providers' performance on specific measures of quality and efficiency. The purpose of VBP models is to provide incentives or payment based on quality measures with the assumption that improved quality improves health outcomes and reduces costs to the insurer. Examples of measures or metrics include patient satisfaction, chronic disease management, evidence-based care process completion, outcomes, and reduction in costs or at least a slowdown in rise of costs. For example, a payer may set benchmark or performance targets for 10 diabetes clinical quality measures or a percentage of the population having received breast or colon cancer screenings.

Payment can be in the form of bonus payments or direct incentives or reimbursement for achieving all or some of the measures. The amounts vary among the programs but are usually above the FFS reimbursement for services rendered. Some payers offer reimbursement at higher FFS levels but withhold a percentage until cost and quality targets are achieved.

Occasionally, payers will attempt to utilize a withhold from basic reimbursement until targets are achieved. The incentive is to force physicians to achieve the value-added goals prior to earning normal reimbursement. Physicians generally perceive this as a negative incentive since they have to perform additional work without additional reward.

Programs typically incorporate a physician report card to provide comparisons of the physician's and practice's performance. Data from these report cards can be used in payer physician network directories to provide additional information for patients selecting physicians.

Private Payer Initiatives

What began as P4P programs a decade ago, value-based programs continue to evolve as private payers implement different incentives, metrics, and models as they learn from earlier programs or competitors' programs. Goals are often similar to the National Committee for Quality Assurance's (NCQA's) Healthcare Effectiveness Data and Information Set (HEDIS) quality metrics. Initially, the programs evaluated physicians and practices on at least two criteria:

1. Presence of infrastructure or care delivery systems to support quality care. For example, an electronic health record (EHR) is in place and used to record and analyze patient care data.

2. Providers follow treatment plans and processes that are consistent with accepted quality indicators or clinical best practices. For example, the practice consistently reminds diabetic patients to have annual foot and eye exams. This criterion emphasizes recording the completion of specific activities and was often described as "pay to report."

More recent and sophisticated VBP programs include clinical outcome and patient experience measures, increasing the shift to pay for value. An example of an outcome measure is HbA1c < 8.0 percent for a population of diabetic patients. Programs may also incorporate cost efficiencies or utilization management, such as reduction in unnecessary tests, emergency room visits, or hospitalizations.

The following are a few examples of private-payer VBP initiatives:

- Humana's Provider Quality Rewards program is based on nine HEDIS measures for breast, colorectal, glaucoma, and nephropathy screening, and diabetes metrics including A1c control. It engages smaller practices with less sophisticated systems using historical practice data and providing rewards for improved quality over baseline scores. In its first year (2010), nearly $10 million was distributed to physician practices as incentives and rewards. More advanced practices can participate in medical home programs under which incentive payments are based on care coordination improvements and increasing patient engagement in disease management.[4]

- UnitedHealthcare in Illinois reviewed historical data and graded physicians on quality and efficiency. Physicians achieving United's goals received a 5 percent boost on their contracted rate for all services and received a star for each category in the payer's physician directory. Value-based contracting will grow to 50–70 percent of physicians in network by 2015.[5]

- Blue Cross Blue Shield of Minnesota is also shifting emphasis to prevent illness rather than treating chronic and acute illnesses and including payments based on value determined by total cost of care and outcome measurement. It has shifted to longer-term contracts to build relationships with goals of lowering costs and improving quality and is working toward increasing transparency and sharing of data.[6]

- HealthPartners programs operating in the upper Midwest withhold 1 to 5 percent of providers' revenue, which is returned to physicians based on achieving quality, satisfaction, and efficiency targets.[7]

Private Payer's New Reimbursement Models

The Government Accountability Office found the following common themes after evaluating private payer programs that reimbursed physicians in new models: "Measuring performance and making payments at the physician-group level, rather than the individual patient level; using a standard set of metrics; tying financial incentives to benchmarks as opposed to gauging performance relative to peers; and paying incentives soon after the performance period ends."[8]

CMS's Medicare Value-Based Initiatives

The Centers for Medicare & Medicaid Services (CMS) has introduced several Medicare programs to begin the shift toward paying for value. The agency's programs have followed this concept:

> *The concept of value-based health care purchasing is that buyers should hold providers of health care accountable for both cost and quality of care. Value-based purchasing brings together information on the quality of health care, including patient outcomes and health status, with data on the dollar outlays going towards health. It focuses on managing the use of the health care system to reduce inappropriate care and to identify and reward the best-performing providers. This strategy can be contrasted with more limited efforts to negotiate price discounts, which reduce costs but do little to ensure that quality of care is improved.[9]*

Many of Medicare's reimbursement demonstration programs and initiatives were introduced or required by the Patient Protection and Affordable Care Act (PPACA), but several were in place prior to the act's passage. The CMS Center for Medicare & Medicaid Innovation (CMMI) has also been the source of several specific new payment and service delivery models defined by Congress through the PPACA and other legislation. CMMI initiatives include primary care transformation, accountable care, and bundled payment demonstration programs.

"Meaningful Use"

CMS's meaningful use requirements were a first step in incentive programs requiring physicians to show implementation and use of an EHR in the practice by reporting e-prescription and medication reconciliation activity, tracking quality measures and chronic conditions, using clinical decision support tools, and recording patient vitals, diagnoses, and smoking conditions. Complying with meaningful use requirements also showed the capability to track and record various activities, processes, and data needs that become the foundation for additional CMS initiatives and requirements. For this reason, physician's compliance with meaningful use can be a first factor in physician incentive plans.

The incentive payment, after a provider has shown meaningful use of a certified EHR technology, can equal 75 percent of a physician's total Medicare allowable with annual caps. Beginning in 2015, professionals not demonstrating meaningful use of an EHR will face reductions in their Medicare fee schedule reimbursement rates. The penalty will equal 1 percent in 2015, 2 percent in 2016, and 3 percent in 2017 and each subsequent year. As of April 2013, eligible professionals (EPs) and hospitals had received nearly $13 billion from the CMS as part of the Meaningful Use EHR incentive program.[10]

Physician Quality Reporting System

The Physician Quality Reporting System (PQRS) is the Medicare quality reporting program for providers to track and submit their patient care data to a system that will help them evaluate and improve the quality of care they provide. Providers were initially rewarded to document and report that they had completed defined steps in quality measures for many chronic diseases and episodic care along with adoption and use of EHRs and e-prescribing. Each physician or administrator should review and understand each measure specification to identify those applicable to the practice and the means to reach the expected targets.

What began as a voluntary reporting system with incentive payments will penalize providers who don't participate; a 1.5 percent penalty will be applied to the practice's total estimated Medicare Part B allowed charges by 2015 and a 2 percent penalty in 2016. PQRS data will also be used in Physician Compare, the Medicare provider rating method available to beneficiaries. Physician Compare will report quality measures reported under PQRS along with assessment of care coordination, patient outcomes, patient experience, and efficiency of care.

Many private payers have implemented programs ranking physicians based on quality and cost-effectiveness. Anthem's Blue Precision and UnitedHealthcare's UnitedHealth Premium are just two examples. The information is used as a tool to encourage enrollees to select physicians that meet the insurer's ideals.

Value-Based Reimbursement Modifier

A value-based payment modifier (VBPM) under the Medicare Physician Fee Schedule offers differential payments to physicians or groups of physicians based on the quality of care furnished compared to the cost of care. "CMS will use PQRS quality measures, total per-capita cost measures, and the per-capita cost measures for patients with four specific conditions to determine quality and cost scores under the program." As stated in the PPACA, the VBPM must be budget-neutral, which means that any upward payment adjustments awarded for higher quality and lower costs must be balanced by downward payment adjustments for providing lower quality at higher costs.

The modifier will initially apply to physician group practices with 100 or more EPs in 2015 based on reported data from 2013. The modifier will be applied beginning in 2017 to all physicians who will bill Medicare under the Physician Fee Schedule.

Groups will receive rating of high, average, and low depending on position relative to the national mean for quality and cost scores. Upward payment adjustment to be distributed to high performers will be determined after calculating the downward payment adjustment for low performers. Groups that don't participate in the PQRS will be penalized up to 1.5 percent of Part B payments starting January 1, 2015.[11]

Patient-Centered and Primary Care Initiatives

Many health policy analysts and healthcare leaders believe that one of the keys to driving down healthcare costs is to start with primary care. By increasing care management at the primary care provider level, the early identification and improved management of chronic diseases and increased rate of preventive care services will result in an expected drop in hospitalizations and readmissions with lower expenses.

To gain these benefits, payers are encouraging primary care providers through several initiatives and incentives. Primary care initiatives take many names and forms, from advanced primary care to patient-centered primary care and medical homes.

Primary care emphasis goes hand in hand with the concept of patient-centered care, which is defined in many ways. The Agency for Healthcare Research and Quality (AHRQ), an agency of the U.S. Department of Health and Human Services, refers to patient-centered care as a move away from disease-centered care. The AHRQ now recommends moving toward encouraging patients to "become active participants in their own care and receive services designed to focus on their individual needs and preferences, in addition to advice and counsel from health professionals."[12] A practice can become patient centered by adopting the principles without seeking formal certification.

Patient centeredness is defined according to activities that put the patient in the center of care:

- A process is in place to ensure that patients receive lab, radiology, and other medical results regardless of normal or abnormal outcomes;

- Patients and caregivers are involved in a formal advisory capacity (i.e., patient and family advisory council);

- A mission or vision statement that explicitly includes the term "patient-centered care";

- Providers ask patients if there are external factors (i.e., nonmedical/clinical issues) that make it difficult to take care of their health needs;

- Care is coordinated for the patient instead of relying on the patient to schedule referrals, tests, and so on;

- Patients and caregivers directly participate with staff in developing mutually agreed-upon treatment plans; and

- Patient access is prioritized by offering same-day appointments or as soon as possible and additional hours of operation or e-mail and phone access.[13]

Care Management and Coordination

Care management or coordination is seen as an important factor in improving patient health and reducing costs by increasing patient contact and education, more intensively managing chronic conditions, and coordinating care between providers. There are several initiatives from private and public payers to encourage care management or coordination through additional reimbursement to cover additional costs related to intensive patient management. The medical home concept is one of the care management incentives.

Johns Hopkins developed a program called Guided Care that relies on nurse care coordinators and is being adopted by other healthcare entities. Cigna launched the Collaborative Accountable Care initiative in 2008 with the specific goals of increasing patient access to reduce unnecessary emergency room visits, hospital discharge coordination, and patient education and coaching to improve patient self-management. Cigna sponsored hiring nurse care coordinators to handle many of these tasks.

The CMS Comprehensive Primary Care Initiative is a multipayer initiative fostering collaboration between public and private healthcare payers to strengthen primary care. Medicare will work with commercial and state health insurance plans and offer bonus payments to primary care doctors who better coordinate care for their patients.

In addition, CMS introduced two new Transitional Care Management services codes to reimburse for care coordination in the 30 days following a Medicare beneficiary's discharge from an inpatient hospital, skilled nursing facility, community mental health center, or outpatient hospital observation services.

Medical Homes

Medical homes are care delivery methods characterized as "a physician practice and patient partnership that provides accessible, interactive, family focused, coordinated and comprehensive care."[14] Four organizations offer practices patient-centered

EXHIBIT 4.1 ■ Medical Home Reimbursement Methods

FFS plus care coordination fee	40.7%
Full risk capitation	18.5%
Pay for performance (quality and clinical incentive payments)	26.0%
Episode of care payment	7.4%

Source: *Guide to Medical Home Reimbursement*, Healthcare Intelligence Network, Sea Girt, N.J., 2010, www.hin.com, 888.446.3530, p. 12–13.

medical home (PCMH) status or certification: the Accreditation Association for Ambulatory Health Care, NCQA, URAC, as well as The Joint Commission. NCQA offers a widely accepted certification program for practices that want to be recognized as PCMHs. The foundations of a PCMH are:

1. "Whole-person care is patient centered with emphasis on the patient's experience;

2. Personal clinician provides first contact, continuous, comprehensive care;

3. Care is coordinated or integrated across the health care system;

4. Team-based care."[15,16]

Reimbursement Incentives for Care Coordination and Medical Homes

CMS's Comprehensive Primary Care Initiative is intended to encourage PCMHs and practices planning to achieve certification. Medicare will work with commercial and state health insurance plans and offer monthly bonus payments to primary care physicians (PCPs) who better coordinate care for their patients.[17]

Several private payers and state Medicaid programs recognize and reward medical homes through care coordination fees, increased payment for evaluation and management (E&M) services, or quality and outcome bonuses. The most common method of reimbursing medical homes (Exhibit 4.1) is a care coordination fee paid as a per member per month (PMPM) amount. The care coordination fee recognizes the extra resource requirements for care coordination. The PMPM amount varies depending on level of NCQA certification and can range from $3 in a Medicaid program to an average of $20 for a Medicare program under CMS's Comprehensive Primary Care Initiative. Other payers increase the reimbursement for physicians in medical homes by a set percentage, either for all services or just E&M and immunization services.

Some payers are using a mix of reimbursement methods to split the physicians' incentives among several factors, including quality, care management, and individual services. WellPoint's PCMH initiatives used a mix of reimbursements such as FFS as the base payment, a PMPM care coordination fee, and a P4P incentive based on quality and cost or utilization factors. Some of WellPoint's programs used enhanced payments for E&M services or for physicians in PCMHs achieving higher-level certification.[18] WellPoint increased reimbursement to primary care providers by an average of 10 percent for practices adopting "patient-centered practice principles."[19]

Capital District Physicians' Health Plan in New York uses a payment system that is 10 percent based on FFS, 63 percent by capitation adjusted for patient severity, and 27 percent as bonus payment based on improvements in patient satisfaction, value, quality, and cost.[20] CareFirst BlueCross BlueShield increased fees by 12 percent for physicians participating in care coordination and offers bonuses that could total 20 percent, based on achieving quality score measures, electronic prescribing, use of EHRs, and targets for reducing health costs.[21]

Shared Savings and Accountable Care Organizations

Shared savings programs allow participants to keep part of the savings realized by the payer for specific services or the total cost of care per beneficiary or population. The federal government first considered allowing gainsharing in the late 2000s, encouraging hospitals and providers to reduce costs through product and supply standardization, application of efficient treatment protocols, and improved care coordination. Shared savings programs include incentives for physicians to unite efforts with hospitals and other service providers in order to succeed in improving value. These programs provide new incentives and rewards.

Accountable care organizations (ACOs) are frequently used by CMS and several private payers as part of their shared savings programs to encourage multiple provider organizations to unite in a single entity to share accountability and rewards. The ACOs are expected to improve their patient population's health by coordinating inpatient and outpatient services and investing in infrastructure and redesigned care processes. The requirements to be an ACO vary by payer, but all are eligible to receive payments for shared savings after they meet quality performance and risk-adjusted standards. Services are reimbursed based on FFS, so there is no downside risk.[22]

Although the Medicare's ACO program receives most of the attention, several private payers have implemented similar programs. Cigna's Collaborative Accountable Care initiative provides financial incentives to physician groups and integrated delivery systems to improve the quality and efficiency of care for patients in commercial open-access benefit plans. The initiative is aimed at managing at-risk populations and includes incentives for hospitals to notify physicians of patient admissions to ensure transition-of-care after discharge. Cigna offers up-front payments to encourage extension of medical practice hours or purchase of information technology systems to support care coordination and e-prescribing.[23]

Hawaii Medical Service Association (HMSA), Hawaii's largest insurer, entered in a shared-savings agreement with the state's biggest health system, Hawaii Pacific Health, and "puts 50 percent of the hospital's annual pay increases over the five-year contract term dependent on achieving both quality improvement and cost savings thresholds." HMSA's physician payments already factor in HEDIS scores and other quality measures.[24]

The keys to succeeding under shared savings incentives are understanding who the patient population is and how to achieve the quality performance benchmarks. Understanding the population includes knowing patient demographics and tracking the total services they are receiving (pharmacy, all physicians, hospitals, and ancillary services), which requires communication among the participating entity (ACO), payer, and other providers.

The CMS quality performance standards for ACOs include:

- Patient/caregiver experience (7 measures) – gathered in the CG-CAHPS (Clinician and Group Consumer Assessment of Healthcare Providers and Systems) patient survey;

- Care coordination/patient safety (6 measures) including hospital readmission rate, hospital admissions for COPD (chronic obstructive pulmonary disease) and heart failure, and EHR meaningful use and medication reconciliation;

- Preventive health (8 measures) including immunization and vaccination rates, and health screening completion; and

- At-risk population determined by quality metrics for diabetes, hypertension, ischemic vascular disease, heart failure, and coronary artery disease.[25]

It will be up to each ACO to determine how to distribute the shared savings payment among participating hospitals, physicians, and other providers. Even without the CMS requirement that the ACO be managed by a separate entity, many health systems have set up a separate physician–hospital organization or hired a third-party administrator to manage the payments. This separate party contributes a sense of shared governance and trust. Distribution to physicians within participating medical groups will depend on the group's compensation plan and the incentives it includes.

Risk-Shifting Initiatives

Part of this changing reimbursement methodology is the trend toward shifting more risk onto the providers. The general theme of risk shifting is to replace FFS reimbursement (pay for volume) with a flat preset payment for a service or per enrollee. If providers' costs are below the payment, then they keep the extra. If costs are higher, then the provider(s) absorbs the loss. Under risk agreements, providers frequently purchase stop-loss or other insurance to help minimize the risk.

Payers have tried shifting risk under capitation, which became widespread in the 1980s and early 1990s. When a backlash ensued, partially because the emphasis was solely on cost containment not quality, the frequency of capitation reimbursement declined except in a few markets. At-risk types of arrangements are back, but they are in the form of bundled payments and what are now called global payments. These payment methods now incorporate quality along with financial metrics based on utilization.

Risk-shifting initiatives have been initiated or reintroduced by public and private payers. Providers under such programs will be rewarded for cost-effectiveness while maintaining quality and experience of care or improving outcomes. Some of these programs are so new, participating entities are still struggling with how to distribute risk and reward between hospitals, physicians, and other providers involved in the included services. Physician compensation methodologies need to incorporate appropriate incentives. Examples of risk-shifting reimbursement systems, in order of increasing risk, include:

- Case rate;
- Bundled payments; and
- Capitation and global payments.

Case Rate

Case rate payments are fixed, pre-established payment for a specific case. Each case is paid the same rate regardless of complexity. The most frequent examples are for obstetric and orthopedic services. Obstetricians are paid one rate for deliveries, which includes expected pre- and postnatal care.

A new model is the Evidence-informed Case Rate (ECR®) under the Prometheus Payment model developed by the Health Care Incentives Improvement Institute. ECR is a payment budget established for all providers who will interact with the patient for a given condition, including the hospital, physicians, laboratory, pharmacy, and rehabilitation facility. The rate is based on expected costs adjusted for the patient's age, gender, and other demographic and risk factors. For physicians, 10 percent of the case rate payment is held back in a performance contingency fund. The fund is used to reward efficient use of evidence-based treatment within the agreed-upon rate, with optimal referral and collaboration efforts. Unfortunately, the formula is complex and proprietary, making it difficult for providers to predict the expected payment amount.[26]

Bundled Payments

Bundled payments are single payments to cover multiple services related to an applicable episode of care. An episode of care includes a hospitalization or procedure and the related services provided prior to admission and following discharge. The goal is to encourage collaboration of inpatient or outpatient hospital services, physicians, and post-acute care and other providers to reduce costs while maintaining quality. Since payment is less than the sum of previous payments, the entities must reduce costs through standardization, managing length of stay, coordinating transfer of care, ensuring that discharge planning is followed through, or other steps. To reduce readmissions and other adverse consequences, services are tracked for a period after hospitalization or an outpatient procedure. Bundled payments are opportunities for payers and providers to manage a patient population, coordinate information sharing and efforts, and manage costs without the complexity and amount of risk of capitated contracts. However, this payment mechanism only addresses episodic care and not the long-term and chronic disease management care that drives a large percentage of U.S. healthcare costs.

Not only are payers shifting more risk to providers, but they also shift the responsibility of how the payment is distributed among providers. Hospitals typically receive the payment since they have the responsibility of tracking the different services to complete a care episode and are more capable of distributing payments to other providers.

One of Medicare's bundled payment demonstration programs was the Acute Care Episode program, which included cardiac and orthopedic inpatient procedures. Participating organizations needed to achieve hospital and physician quality metrics prior to receiving shared savings distribution.[27] A more recent CMS initiative is Bundled Payments for Care Improvement, which offers four models with different requirements.

An example of a private payer's bundled payment program is UnitedHealthcare's pilot for treatment of breast, colon, and lung cancers. Payment was based on volume of drugs administered, revenue the group would make on drug expense margins, and a "case management fee to reflect the time and resources that the oncologist's office spends in managing the patient relationship."[28] Geisinger Health System in Pennsylvania developed bundled payment programs for elective coronary artery bypass, perinatal care, bariatric surgery, and other services.

Capitation and Global Payments

Capitation, once in vogue in the 1980s and 1990s, is seeing a return, although in sometimes modified forms. *Capitation* is defined as "payment for the obligation to furnish all or part (e.g., physician professional services only) of care for a given population of patients typically paid on a per beneficiary (member) per month basis (PMPM). Payment amount is adjusted for patient demographics, including age, sex, and health status."[29] If costs for patient care amount to less than the payment, providers keep the difference. If, however, healthcare costs exceed the payment, doctors make up the difference out of their own pockets.

The goal of capitation or global payments is to eliminate incentives for volume and encourage utilization management. Capitation in the 1990s stumbled because there weren't incentives for quality or patient satisfaction and medical practices did not have the data capabilities to truly manage patient population and risk. NCQA developed HEDIS to ensure that quality and satisfaction were included in how managed care organizations operated and reimbursed medical practices.

Capitation is typically only directed toward one provider/practice, but there are many types of capitation from primary care specific, specialty specific, contact capitation, and so forth. Global payments account for either all patient care or for a specific group of services delivered to a patient population, including outpatient physician, ancillary, hospital services, and prescription drugs. Since global payments cover more services than physicians provide, payments are frequently directed toward integrated health systems or ACOs.[30]

Other features that may be included in capitation or global payment systems include:

- Risk sharing between healthcare provider and insurance entity;
- Health status adjustments based on population risk factors;
- Enhanced integrative healthcare systems, including data sharing;
- Risk corridors where provider and insurance entity establish floors and ceilings to the amount of risk shared;
- Reinsurance or stop-loss options to mitigate risk margins for providers and insurers; and
- Financial incentives tied to quality performance measures.

Blue Cross Blue Shield of Massachusetts (BCBS) introduced global payments in its Alternative Quality Contract with primary care and multispecialty practices. The annual global budget is based on each participating group's previous PMPM spending. BCBS provides quality-based performance bonuses and regular reports on spending, service use, and quality of care. Groups are paid FFS during the year and all medical care payments, both within group and out of group, are deducted against the global budget. At year end, BCBS reconciles with each group, paying any money left in global budget or "recouping" what was spent overbudget. The quality aspect uses 64 measures – 32 for inpatient and 32 for outpatient care – covering process of care, outcomes, and patient experience. Participants must receive the minimum quality score. If the highest score is achieved, the bonus can be 10 percent of total medical spending with 5 percent from ambulatory quality measures and 5 percent for inpatient quality measures.[31]

To succeed under bundled and global payments, providers must understand three factors:

1. **Member reconciliation or patient attribution.** This measure is defined as the specific patient population that the provider is responsible for. Providers must know the number of members, demographics, and risk adjustment of the population to fully understand the risk of the contract. The amount of risk will also depend on whether or not patients are explicitly assigned to the provider entity and how patients' choice of providers and services is managed through a referral requirement.

2. **Scope of services or benefits that are covered under the contract.** Does it include just office visits or minor procedures and hospital visits, pharmaceutical and ancillary services? Services and benefits must be clearly defined in the contract.

3. **Handling of out-of-network care.** Will the patient, provider, or insurer cover out-of-network costs and under what circumstances?

Physician performance and incentive programs under these reimbursement mechanisms must emphasize population health management and cost management, including limiting the number of unnecessary referrals, procedures, and diagnostic services. Practice executives must watch for adverse patient selection or incorporate the number of higher-risk patients in incentive systems.[32]

Physician Compensation and Risk-Based Contracting. Medical groups that participate in risk-shifting initiatives, particularly capitation and global payments, should ensure that physician compensation incentives align with the financial realities and reimbursement incentives of the risk contracts. Capitation contracts can penalize practices with compensation formulas that encourage high productivity. New reimbursement incentives that are based on quality and value should be matched by similar compensation formulas. For example, according to a survey of 21 large, multispecialty groups participating in risk contracts, groups with more revenue from risk-based contracts had a slightly higher share of physician compensation dependent on performance measures: 5 percent for specialists and 7–12 percent for PCPs. Most of the groups expected to change their physician compensation calculation in the next two years to match the predicted shift from FFS revenue to revenue from shared savings, pay for performance, and global capitation. The responding groups received an average of 25 percent of revenue from global capitation contracts and 9 percent from partial capitation or shared risk. Most had more than 440 physicians, and many had affiliated health plans.[33]

Compensation Models and Value-Based Incentives

Although currently a small percentage of total reimbursement, value-based payments (VBPs) and other new reimbursement models are expected to increase over time as a means of reducing overall healthcare costs while ensuring that patient health is

EXHIBIT 4.2 ■ Differences between Traditional FFS and Value-Based Reimbursement

Feature	Traditional FFS	Value-Based Methods
Payment	Retrospective reimbursement	Prospective payment with rewards and penalties
Risk	None	Low: Shared savings and gainsharing
		High: Bundled and global payments
Quality of care	Assumed	Measured and reported with rewards and penalties
Provider integration	Not required/optional	Hospital, physician, ancillary providers
Data reporting	None required	Cost and quality metrics, utilization, and patient satisfaction

Source: John P. Schmitt, PhD, and Robert W. Keen, Esq., "Payer Contracting: Strategies to Boost Your Bottom Line while Preparing for Value-Based Contracts." Reliance Consulting Group, MGMA webinar, October 11, 2012.

improved by the services provided. Even if a group is not currently receiving VBPs, it should consider modifying the compensation methodology to include incentives for quality, outcomes, and patient satisfaction. This will prepare the group and its physicians for a value-based environment in the future.

Also, a new trend among payers is to publish physicians' standing on quality and cost benchmarks to patients or referring physicians or at least use the data in providing star or premium ratings in physician network directories. Medicare uses PQRS results in its Physician Compare listing. Ensuring good standing under payers' metrics will increase patient and referral selection. An incentive system will also align physicians with organizational missions of providing quality care and ensuring patient satisfaction.

Exhibit 4.2 highlights the differences between FFS and value-based reimbursement. Physician compensation incentives must follow the shift in culture and processes that must occur to succeed under value-based payment.

The difficulty is in how to incorporate the incentives in a physician compensation plan while still in a largely FFS environment that emphasizes volume. Medical practices find themselves in a conflicting world for a while, similar to when they received mixed income and therefore mixed incentives from FFS and capitation. Currently, FFS still predominates in most markets but if it shrinks compared to increasing value-based reimbursement, there will be a difficult period of balancing the productivity incentive to maintain revenue under the old system while the new reimbursement is driving different incentives. It will be important for medical practices to develop flexible compensation formulas to adjust to the changing incentives over time.

These new reimbursement systems may not easily translate into physician compensation formulas. Also, adverse incentives must be considered and addressed. For example, capitation limited to a group of PCPs in some cases increased the number of referrals to other providers in order to shift costs of patient care to other physicians. Payers' withhold systems may encourage additional volume to make up for the withhold amount. Plan developers must identify the desired behavior to succeed under the reimbursement system and how the behavior can be encouraged and rewarded. Compensation plans must be flexible enough to allow adjustments for differences in payers' systems and their changing incentives. As mentioned earlier in this chapter, keeping the compensation plan simple and understandable won't be easy.

Incentive plans, like the total compensation plan, must also be customized to the practice. Each group is different in terms of the marketplace, reimbursement incentives, and the culture, goals, and objectives. Therefore, each group must identify priorities in the incentive plan, desired behavior that should be encouraged and rewarded, and how much of total compensation to include at risk or as an incentive. Even within one delivery model, medical homes, there will be a variety of compensation formulas.

Regardless of the payers' quality and utilization management incentive plans, accurate patient data is critical, and in many cases, help from actuarial experts would be beneficial. In addition, there are ways to mitigate or manage risk to some extent with stop-loss insurance. Each medical group must decide how it is going to absorb losses and/or distribute positive earnings. Depending on the circumstances, some practices will treat losses or bonuses as a group issue and allocate them as a function of compensation cash available and distribute under the regular compensation plan. This works well when the potential bonus or loss is fairly immaterial in relation to total compensation. In other cases, the group may decide to allocate all or a portion of losses/bonuses down to an individual physician level. This may not be a material factor if the risk of loss to the individual physician is fairly low. However, if the risk of loss to the individual physician is significant, then this could have adverse ramifications relating to physician retention. The decision to accept a reimbursement contract with the potential of losses should be a group decision. In these cases, many groups decide to absorb all or the majority of losses at a group level and restrict the amount of loss that can be transferred to individual physicians. All of these decisions will be dependent on specific situations and could change from year to year as circumstances change.

Steps in Incentive Plan Development

The first step in developing a successful value-based incentive system is for physicians to see the importance of change themselves, according to Randy Cook, MPH,

FACMPE, president/CEO, AmpliPHY Physician Services. Physicians must recognize the need to change clinical practices and organizational culture to improve the quality of patient care and experience. Most physicians already believe in quality of care; implementing a new compensation method introduces the means of tracking care quality and rewarding it. There is even more incentive for physicians if reimbursement is based on the quality of patients' care.

With physician buy-in to the process, the following steps should be taken to develop a value-based incentive compensation plan:

1. Select the value-based metrics;

2. Determine individual, team, and organizational measures and incentives;

3. Establish the size and source of incentive pool;

4. Determine the weighting of measures;

5. Decide if the reward is to be based on target achievement, improvement, or maintenance; and

6. Identify the incentive payment mechanism.

Selecting Value-Based Metrics

For medical practices not currently under new reimbursement programs, incentives should be traced to the mission and vision statements along with goals and objectives of the compensation planning process. If the mission and vision of the organization include statements such as "providing the best quality of care," "ensuring the highest customer satisfaction," or "we are a patient-centered practice," then quality and patient satisfaction should be measured and included in the compensation methodology. Achieving quality and satisfaction goals can enable a practice to market itself to patients and payers as truly offering quality of care and satisfaction, perhaps providing a competitive edge.

For medical practices currently receiving or soon to receive payments from new reimbursement programs, along with organizational goals and values, the key is to "follow the money." This means identifying the quality metrics, cost measures, and patient experience factors that are used to determine reimbursement or incentive payments. The incentive program, contracts, and provider manuals should be studied to identify which cost and quality measures will be used, and how withholds, bonuses, and risk sharing will be handled. Payers should provide reports on current practice results in the areas that they track and measure to establish base metrics. Payers may also help identify what changes need to be implemented to reach or exceed the expected performance benchmarks. It is important to correctly identify what factors payers are prioritizing and the current practice's standing in order to identify measures and processes to implement for the greatest initial gain.

Many payers set their own priorities, which may be different than those of other payers or Medicare's. Practice executives should review current and future contracts with their major payers to determine which measures are common across many payers or which reimbursement incentives will have the greatest impact on the practice, depending on the current number of patients or amount of revenue from each payer. Start by listing each of the practice's payers and the percentage of revenue received from each payer. Then record the current reimbursement model and future reimbursement plans for each payer. The group may choose to minimize effort toward payers that represent a small percentage of revenue, or work with these payers to utilize metrics the group is already focusing on. For payers that provide a majority of revenue, conduct a careful analysis of the payer's incentives, current quality metrics, and plans for the future. Review the various payers' information and identify common quality metrics.

For help in identifying and comparing quality measures used in your community and others, look at an online tool from the National Quality Forum (NQF). The "Community Tool to Align Measurement" was developed to help providers, communities, and others identify and compare NQF-endorsed measures others are using and what their experience has been. The tool provides insight for those interested in starting or expanding measurement and public reporting in ways that align with others as well as national programs.[34]

The practice should pick three to six measures as a starting point in incentive compensation formulas. Single-specialty practices should select the same measures for all physicians. Multispecialty practices may identify some common measures for all physicians, such as patient satisfaction or EHR utilization. Other measures should be specialty or department specific. If physicians participate in the selection process, they will have more buy-in to the incentives and target benchmarks. Sources for information on quality metrics are listed in Appendix A. Examples of value-based, quality, and performance metrics are listed in Exhibit 4.3.

Keep in mind that the practice does not have to commit to the same criteria forever. The intent is to encourage and reward behavior toward improvement in patient satisfaction, outcomes, and value. Targets shift over time depending on internal and external goals. As goals in any category are achieved, the targets can be changed or new criteria introduced. Links to previous criteria can be maintained with a small percentage of incentive compensation or just through the physician performance reviews.

Organizational goals of increasing patient satisfaction will drive selection of patient satisfaction, access, and experience benchmarks that are meaningful and measureable. Goals to increase quality, such as improving diabetes care management, will lead to selection of quality and chronic disease management measures. Objectives to

EXHIBIT 4.3 ■ Value-Based Metrics List

These are the general categories and examples of the criteria that may be used in a payer's incentive programs and could be incorporated in physician compensation and incentive plans. This list is not meant to be comprehensive.

Access: waiting times, second or third next available appointment, utilization of e-mail or e-visit patient communication, hours of availability

Process: hemoglobin A1c testing twice annually, implement drug formulary checks, coordinated and documented patient transition, patient provided with care plan

Outcomes: percentage of patients with reduced A1c, percentage of patients enrolled in smoking cessation programs, high blood pressure control, lipid and LDL control

Patient experience: patient satisfaction, how well providers communicated, eliciting patient's participation in shared decision making, patient health status or functional status

Care coordination and patient safety: physician qualifies for EHR program incentive; medication reconciliation, patient falls and screening for future fall risk, catheter-associated urinary tract infection, team participation and support

Preventive health: vaccinations, influenza immunization rate, blood pressure measurement, cancer screening, tobacco use screening

Utilization and resource demand: emergency room visits, readmissions, unnecessary diagnostic imaging or laboratory tests, number of referrals, generic prescription rate, use of standardized medical equipment, supplies, and order sets.

Participation and scores in current quality- and outcome-based programs:

- HEDIS scores, NCQA
- CMS's EHR Meaningful Use
- CMS's PQRS
- Medical home certification

Specialist metrics examples:

- Specialty-specific quality metrics and treatment protocols;
- Referring physician satisfaction surveys including timeliness and quality of response;
- Care coordination with referring physician and other providers;
- Compliance with evidence-based medicine protocols;
- Post-acute-care management;
- Number of unnecessary readmissions;
- Medication reconciliation;
- Discharge planning and care plan development;
- Patient access in terms of appointment availability or other factor; and
- Patient satisfaction or experience.

modify behavior within the practice, such as completing charts in a timely manner or participating in practice administration, might be considered. A payer's incentive to reduce emergency room visits or hospital readmissions can be met with incentives to increase patient access or to more intensively managed care coordination and patient transition. Patient-centered practices, including medical homes, may select factors for encouraging and measuring care coordination, team participation, and patient experience. Part of the patient experience that should be recognized is including patients in self-management and care plans.

Practices receiving reimbursement through shared savings and bundled or global payments should consider including metrics related to care coordination, utilization management, and cost management since these are factors in determining reimbursement, along with quality factors. Appropriate metrics include number of unnecessary emergency room visits or hospital readmissions, number of diagnostic imaging and other tests, utilizing standard medical equipment and supplies, number of referrals, discharge care plan development, and so on. Quality and outcome measures used by Medicare's ACO shared savings determination should also be considered.

Global payments drive population health management incentives as were first experienced under capitation in the 1990s. Incentive plans should reduce the push for volume that underlies productivity-based compensation. Some groups found more success under capitation by basing a higher percentage of compensation on salary or emphasizing patient panel size that can now include patient risk and acuity adjustments.

The compensation committee and physicians should select several criteria and evaluate which measures to include based on several criteria including:

- What is the source of data for the measure? Is it external, from payers, and can their data be trusted? Does the practice management or EHR system currently track data? Do changes need to be made to ensure that appropriate information is recorded in current systems? Can internal data be cross-checked with external data?

- What is the desired behavior needed to achieve targets for the measure?

- Are the measures understandable?

- Are the measures meaningful to the physician? Will they capture the interest of the physician from a clinical quality point of view?

- Are the measures objective or subjective? Objective measures should be emphasized.

- Are the metrics within the physicians' control or are they dependent on team, department, or organizational activities?

- Can the data be captured and reported in a timely manner? The more frequently that data can be reported, the quicker physicians will see their status and relate it to their behavior and compensation.

- Do the measures align with the mission, vision, culture, and reimbursement?

- Can steps toward achieving the target or goal be tracked and reported?

- Will the impact of achieving the goal be measured?

Once the selection of metrics is reduced to those that the practice and physicians understand and can track, then it should be determined which three to six criteria should be included in the compensation formula. Start with a mix of criteria that are relatively easy to attain and some that will drive behavioral and organizational change toward needed goals. Implementing patient satisfaction incentives are a good first step for medical groups not currently receiving value-based reimbursement or incentives. CMS's EHR meaningful use requirements are additional factors to consider.

Identifying Data Sources. Once the measures are selected, metrics must be determined and baseline data obtained. Look at comparative data for the measures to see how the group's physicians are doing compared to each other and external data. Benchmarking to external data will provide goals toward improved performance with other medical groups. Even if the group is doing well compared to external numbers, there is always a possibility of setting higher goals as long as the targets are reasonable. If goals are perceived to be out of reach, they tend to be ignored.

Patient satisfaction goals are frequently a first choice for groups since they can be applicable to all practices whether there are external incentives or not. Several tools are available in the marketplace that offer nationwide or regional comparative reports for benchmarking practice performance. They are also objective sources of data, although based on the subjective responses of patients, if enough responses are received.

For example, MGMA-ACMPE partnered with SullivanLuallin Group to build a tool that helps practices assess their current patient satisfaction levels and identify areas of improvement. The tool uses data from the CG-CAHPS survey and can be used to benchmark practice data with nationwide CG-CAHPS and SullivanLuallin data.

The selected survey tool should use CG-CAHPS for numerous reasons:

- Accepted by CMS and other payers;

- Allows comparisons with other clinics/physicians/practices;

- Public access so you know what patients are seeing;

- CMS incentives to participate in the survey; and

- Several versions depending on setting, including PCMH and hospital versions.

Achieving PQRS goals is another example of incentives that can be implemented early in physician incentive programs because of the emphasis on the PQRS. CMS payments will be impacted by PQRS status, and PQRS scores will be used in Medicare's Physician Compare program. Similar information is used by private payers, and scoring well on private and Medicare's quality standards will become an increasing factor in a patient's selection of physicians. Reviewing the PQRS and a private payer's quality measures and expected scores will provide groups with several options for including metrics within the practice.

Performance Reports or Scorecards. Once the measurement criteria are selected, the group should determine scoring mechanisms to track progress toward achieving goals and identify when success in obtained. The scoring mechanism can match payers' reports if appropriate or the group can develop its own. The mechanism, like the measures themselves, should be as objective as possible.

The scoring mechanism and data gathering should be tested in performance reports to demonstrate the group's capability of tracking and reporting the selected criteria and viability of the scoring mechanism. Some practices have found that their EHRs were not able to track the patient health and utilization data to the level required. Business intelligence, data mining, or other additional systems were needed. The comparative reports should show the status of individual physician scores compared with average scores for all of the group's physicians and external benchmark data or the overall goal or target. Internal data should be compared with payer and other external sources to ensure that practice information systems are gathering data in a comparable manner as other sources. There may be a need to modify how internal data is recorded (are providers using the correct EHR fields?) or challenge the external data.

Determining Individual, Team, or Organizational Measures and Incentives

Another decision is to use team-based measures and incentives or limit the measures to an individual physician's behavior. The answer is based on the practice's culture and situation. Individual goals may be easier to implement in the first non-productivity incentive plan since they are reliant on just the physician's behavior. Team measures recognize the valuable role of nursing assistants, care coordinators, and many other employees to achieve the desired goals in patient experience and care management. Also, team measures can match organizational goals of increasing team-oriented behavior, especially with the implementation of team-based patient care. The latter is especially true in medical homes, where the use of nonphysician providers and others is needed to ensure whole-person care. A combination of team-based and individual measures is a viable option for many practices and allows for considerable flexibility in plan design.

Examples of team-based measures include patient experience or satisfaction scores, rates of unnecessary hospital admissions or emergency room visits, and population health measures such as average blood pressure, A1c levels, and LDL levels for all diabetic patients.

Organizational measures will help in aligning physicians toward the idea of being part of a larger organization and their need to align to the organization's mission and goals. Organizational goals include achieving budgetary and other financial goals, achieving PCMH certification or other recognition, receiving shared savings, and so forth.

If team-based measures are used, it is important to include all of the team in the measure and reward system and to provide adequate information and training to ensure team activity and knowledge of the system. It should also be obvious that all members' activities are interdependent and impact the desired outcomes.

The group should consider whether or not team participation becomes a measure in and of itself. This is a subjective measure recorded by employee (team-member) surveys or opinions of medical directors, nursing supervisors, or peers. As such, it should be used with caution, using quality survey tools, measurement based on individual vs. average scores, and limited as a factor in determination of total compensation or incentive.

The value-based payments to physicians can be in the form of bonus or incentive payments. *Bonus payments* are defined as "extra payment beyond salary, benefits, and incentive payments." Bonus payments are seen as rewards for a specific behavior or achieving a specific short-term goal. Examples where a bonus may be applicable include achieving organizational goals like receiving PCMH certification, starting a new service, or receiving the first incentive payment or shared savings from a payer. Bonuses may be used more for team and organizational rewards. Individual incentives can be integrated within the compensation formula for long-term recognition and to encourage and reward long-term behavioral changes. They may be more dependent on individual performance rather than team or organizational performance.

Establishing the Size and Source of the Incentive Pool

The amount of compensation dependent on incentives is closely tied to the source of the incentive money. Groups may choose to limit the incentive fund to reimbursement payments from payers and shared savings distributions or they may choose to fund an incentive pool themselves or use traditional revenue to supplement payers' incentives. It may also be practical to fund the incentive pool from internal and external resources. The choice will depend on the priority of value-based measures and clinical transformation that is desired.

Options for funding the incentive pool include the following:

- The amount of dollars received as a result of **payers' incentive reimbursement** or shared savings.

- The percentage or set dollar amount **withheld internally from the total compensation pool.**

- **Profit available at year end.** As described in chapter 3, the practice should withhold a percentage of the compensation fund in case of unforeseen circumstances. In this example, the remaining amount (around 10 percent) is distributed based on physicians' performance in achieving value-based incentives.

- **The dollar amount or percentage withheld** from individual physician compensation. For example, a physician is eligible for $100,000 compensation based on productivity. Twenty percent is withheld until the physician achieves individual value-based targets. The $20,000 withhold is paid depending on the percentage of targets achieved. This is a less desirable option. Physicians may view it in a more negative light, believing that they've earned the money through their productivity and they shouldn't have to earn it a second time.

- **A combination** of external funding and internally withheld funds.

Incentive reimbursement payments passed directly to the physician(s) increase the link for the physicians between their behavior and the reward. Some incentive payments are solely dependent on physicians while others require team efforts and clinical transformation. However, achieving practice transformation that is necessary to receive most value-based payments requires a complete practice investment. The transformation is expensive, frequently requiring new, large IT investments and hiring additional staff from data analysts to care coordinators. A whole team effort is often required to complete the transformation and achieve the value-based goals. These expenses may have to be funded by additional capital investments, borrowing, existing cash flow, or a combination thereof. Groups may decide to use the additional incentive reimbursement to fund the related infrastructure investments and provide team rewards. Only later will physicians receive the incentive payments.

It's not easy to determine the amount of compensation that should be based on performance measures and is therefore at risk.

Most practices are comfortable with a minimal amount for incentive compensation of 5 percent of total compensation, but at least 10 percent may be needed to truly bring meaning to the incentives and affect physician behavior. If incentive payments approach 10 percent of total reimbursement, then the incentive compensation should be at least 10 percent. Some practices have chosen 20 or 30 percent as an opportunity to ensure complete commitment and recognition to patient quality and outcomes.

EXHIBIT 4.4 ■ Weighting Options for Incentive Measures

Performance or Quality Measure	Incentive Plan	
	Option A	Option B
Patient satisfaction	5%	2%
Active medication lists maintained for 80% of patients	5%	4%
Percentage of diabetic patients screened	5%	7%
Percentage of diabetic patients with reduced A1c	5%	7%

Typically, practices will start at the lower percentages and increase over time as the incentive programs become more comprehensive and physicians are used to dealing with multiple incentives.

Determining the Weighting of Measures

After the total incentive pool or percentage of compensation is determined, the amount available for each of the selected measures needs to be decided. Each factor can receive equal weight and, therefore, amount of the available incentive, or some factors may be considered a higher priority and given more weight (see Exhibit 4.4). The weight or percentage of each criterion will be determined by the priorities of the practice and status of the incentive and reimbursement programs. For example, if a large payer has introduced incentives for diabetes care management, then measures related to diabetes management protocols could be added and prioritized. If patient satisfaction is a group priority, the practice may decide to always link a small percentage of incentives to patient satisfaction since it is an organizational priority, but other measures may be retired after their goals are achieved.

Exhibit 4.4 provides amounts in percentages, but the incentive or bonus payments could also be dollar amounts. Exhibit 4.5 includes examples of two options: incentive payments of set amounts and incentive as a percentage of total compensation. Large health systems may prefer set dollar amounts for achieving specific targets, especially if physicians' compensation is largely salary based. Justin Chamblee, vice president of Coker Group, a healthcare consulting firm, has seen health systems provide non-productivity incentives to physicians in the range of $10,000 to $25,000 for PCPs and $15,000 to $50,000 for specialists.[35] Medical practices usually tie incentives more closely to practice revenue and physician compensation and so use a percentage of either physician compensation or the withhold incentive pool. Keep in mind that a $20,000 incentive will be more meaningful to a PCP earning $200,000 than to a surgical specialist earning $600,000.

Justin Chamblee suggests an additional option for incentive payments using variable rates per work relative value unit (wRVU). As previously described in chapter 3, a compensation per wRVU value is selected by the practice. All or a portion of the

EXHIBIT 4.5 ■ Incentive Compensation Options

	wRVUs	Compensation per wRVU Ratio	Base Compensation			
Established Group Standards	3,800	$39.00	$148,200		P4P Performance Options	
MGMA Examples			Production Compensation	(plus Base)	P4P Pool	Potential Total Compensation
Median	4,500	$39.00	$27,300	$148,200	$12,000	$187,500
75th percentile	6,000	$39.00	$85,800	$148,200	$12,000	$246,000
90th percentile	7,200	$39.00	$132,600	$148,200	$12,000	$292,800
MGMA Examples			Production Compensation	(plus Base)	P4P % of Total Compensation	Potential Total Compensation
Median	4,500	$39.00	$27,300	$148,200	5.0%	$184,275
75th percentile	6,000	$39.00	$85,800	$148,200	5.0%	$245,700
90th percentile	7,200	$39.00	$132,600	$148,200	5.0%	$294,840

value is tied to value-based incentives. Achievement of the goals determines if a physician receives the full rate of compensation per RVU or only a portion. For example, if a wRVU value of $40 is selected by the practice, 15 percent or $6 can be linked to value-based factors. If only 80 percent of the goals are achieved, then the physician is compensated at $38.80 per wRVU. In another option, the whole value of the wRVU ratio can be tied to achieving value-based incentives. In this example, if only 80 percent of the goals are achieved, the compensation per wRVU value becomes $32. This is one way to link productivity and quality in compensation formulas.

Deciding Target Achievement, Improvement, or Maintenance

The next step in developing an incentive compensation system is determining how success is measured and rewards or incentives are distributed. Defining targets or thresholds for quality or satisfaction measures will depend on baseline and benchmark data. For example, if the nationwide satisfaction scores are 85.5 compared with the group's average score of 80, then a target of 85 should be the minimum. A higher target can be set to drive providers toward a higher performance, as long as it is seen as attainable. If internal data show that active medication lists are maintained for only 70 percent of the practice's patients compared to the meaningful use benchmark of more than 80 percent, then the target should be set for at least 80 percent.

Most of the quality and outcomes metrics have specific targets based on payers' quality measures or internal selection. The decision is whether or not rewards are provided only when the target is reached or exceeded or if improvement toward the goal is recognized. For example, only when patient satisfaction scores achieve the goal of 85.0 will the physician be eligible for the incentive payment of 5 percent of compensation. This compares with the option of rewarding a smaller percentage (2 or 3 percent or smaller dollar amount) if the patient satisfaction scores improved since previous reporting periods but did not achieve the target. These two options can be classified as achievement or improvement.

The same incentive formula may include some measures with an all-or-nothing recognition basis while others are rewarded for steps or improvements toward the target.

Measures should also be evaluated for their ongoing value. Some criteria will be retired when the goals are achieved and replaced by other measures. Others may be important enough that incentive payments will continue to maintain the current levels of success or provide opportunities for continuous improvement.

The group may also want to decide whether incentive payments are distributed to physicians only if they achieve expected productivity levels or are independent of the productivity benchmarks. Linking incentive payments to productivity reinforces the ongoing majority of reimbursement from FFS but can provide a conflicted environment between productivity and value-based factors.

Identifying the Incentive Payment Mechanism

Physician performance reports or scorecards should be presented to physicians on a frequent basis – monthly, bimonthly, or not more than quarterly would be ideal if the data are available. The timeliness of the data presentation provides more opportunity for physicians to review their data compared to expectations and understand what needs to change to improve the scores. Some incentive programs were initially established to reconcile annually and didn't allow for behavioral change well into the second year. With lag time in reimbursement and receipt of incentives, it may not be possible to identify the amount of funds available for incentive distribution that frequently, but relative frequency will more directly link the additional payment to the performance.

Groups have found it effective to distribute incentive payments separate from the base compensation method of productivity, salary or equal share. In other words, a separate check or notice of automatic deposit creates more impact and reinforces the link between behavior and payments. Incentive distributions can be shared during annual meetings or assemblies held to celebrate successes related to achieving goals.

Medical practices should also decide whether individual incentive results will be distributed to all participants or privately to individual physicians. There is usually significant motivation for the physician on the low end of the scale to improve, although there may be some political fallout from the publication of poor results. One way to address this is to not publish all results for a short period of time (up to a year) but issue a warning that effective in one year (or whatever time period) the comparisons will be published. This should give poorly performing physicians ample opportunity to improve their scores.

The frequency of incentive or bonus payments will depend on the source of funds. Incentive funds developed by practices setting aside a percentage of net revenue can be distributed quarterly or semi-annually. Incentive pools funded solely by external reimbursement will be distributed after the reimbursement is received. CMS will distribute Medicare ACO shared savings payments after a lengthy calculation. This delayed distribution to medical practices will make it harder for practices to directly link their physicians' behavior to the distribution. Practice executives will have to reinforce incentives and the potential for reward throughout the year.

Incentives and Unforeseen Consequences

It was a FFS, pay-for-volume environment that added to the exponential growth in U.S. healthcare expenditures. Paying per procedure, visit, or hospitalization encouraged, or at least did not discourage, providers to recommend more procedures, visits, and days in the hospital. Now payers are shifting toward emphasizing *value*, defined as improved quality and cost-effective. The effort of healthcare organizations to align physician incentives and compensation with value-based reimbursement can result in unforeseen consequences that must be considered in finalizing physician incentive systems. Each of the various main performance measures can provide adverse consequences, as discussed in the following paragraphs.

Patient satisfaction or experience is a component in many of Medicare's and other payers' new reimbursement initiatives. Since patient satisfaction is a relatively subjective measure, likely based on a patient's mood and health prognosis, its use in physician evaluation and compensation has the potential of being abused by both the patient and the provider. One physician was known to offer free donuts to all patients, which probably helped keep patients in happy moods. The survey tool should be carefully evaluated to ensure that appropriate questions are used to gather data on specific visits or procedures and patient–physician interactions. Try to separate the practice-level experience – related to scheduling, parking, and so on – from the actual physician–patient experience. Surveys are also more effective if provided in a timely manner and are risk-adjusted. A comprehensive instrument like the CG-CAHPS survey provides opportunity to limit patient bias in the results. There should also be a statistically valid number of survey responses to minimize the influence of outlier results.

Patients may demand services that are unnecessary or deny accepted protocols. Providers must include more patient education and participation in care plan development to counter potential dissatisfaction over denied requests.

Some specialists, especially hospital-based physicians, have less contact with patients than PCPs or other specialists, making it more difficult for patients to assess their provider interactions. Some health systems are mitigating this issue by providing photographs of the physicians on their satisfaction surveys.

Patients' health outcomes or health status measures may encourage physicians to "cherry-pick" healthier patients or discharge noncompliant patients and those with greater severity of illness. Two options for reducing these concerns are:

1. Evaluate physicians' patient panels to determine average risk severity compared with the total practice and community population to ensure it is within normal expectations; or

2. Recognize and reward physicians with higher at-risk patient populations.

This second option was utilized by Coast Carolina multispecialty practice in North Carolina. Distribution of shared savings payments will include a factor based on Medicare's Hierarchical Condition Category Risk Adjustment Factor. The higher the average risk adjustment score for a physician's patients, the higher the incentive payment.

Cost and utilization control incentives were part of the downfall of capitation systems. Physicians benefited more under capitation if they referred patients to other physicians or denied or limited services that may have improved health outcomes and that patients believed were needed. Physicians also benefited if their patient panels included more members that they managed by limiting the time per patient. New bundled payments and global capitation have incorporated quality and care coordination incentives to keep providers' eyes and a payer's reimbursement on quality not just cost reduction and maximizing the number of patients.

Bundled payments may cause physicians to counter by recommending or providing more services that are reimbursed outside of the bundled payment or modifying their services to include more higher-reimbursed procedures.[36]

Practice executives should monitor statistics on physicians' rates of tests, procedures, readmissions, and costs per patient along with risk adjustment factors to ensure physicians are within accepted ranges for their patient panel.

Medical groups should monitor physician behavior by tracking these factors and potential consequences. Compensation plans can also be designed to minimize adverse consequences by including several factors in incentive formulas to disperse the impact of any one incentive. Incentives can also encourage and reward physicians with the largest patient population with chronic conditions while maintaining or improving those patients' health statuses.

Compensation plans shouldn't and probably can't be designed to eliminate all potential abuses regardless whether intentional or not. Monitoring and identification of individual physician problems can frequently be addressed by practice administration and physician leadership with the physician on a one-to-one basis.

Incentive Plan Implementation

Implementing incentive compensation should be part of the total compensation plan approval and implementation, discussed in chapter 7. If there is time to prepare for new reimbursement incentives or changing organizational goals, then initially sharing the physician performance reports or scorecards may lead to a desired behavior of achieving organizational value-based goals because of physicians' competitive nature and desire to provide quality care. This also provides physicians with a period to become accustomed to the concept before it affects their compensation. A small percentage of compensation can be placed at risk the following year and over time as the percentage is increased.

After an initial period, the incentive amount should be large enough to gain the physicians' attention but not so large as to create excessive stress or a sense of unfairness leading to a temptation to game the system. The current marketplace is still largely FFS driving incentives toward maintaining volume. As stated earlier, for medical practices joining Medicare's or private payers' incentive or risk-sharing programs, the compensation formula should align incentives and compensation with the reimbursement and incentive systems. Therefore, the amount of compensation at risk under the new incentives should, at a minimum, mirror the percentage of revenue under the new systems. This increases the link between physician behavior and the introduction of new reimbursement methods.

When the health system migrates to greater emphasis on value-based reimbursement, then compensation formulas should parallel or be slightly behind that shift. However, groups can also decide to show commitment to quality and outcome measures by committing a higher percentage of the internal compensation pool toward incentives. The expected improvements in quality and health status can be used to negotiate with payers for higher or additional compensation, especially if cost reductions in total patient care can be confirmed.

End Notes

1. Victoria Stagg Elliott, "3 Steps to Quality Pay for Physicians," *amednews* (July 23, 2012), http://www.ama-assn.org/amednews/2012/07/23/bisa0723.htm (accessed February 14, 2013).

2. Victoria Stagg Elliott, "Physician Employment: Build a Contract That Suits You," *amednews* (January 14, 2013), http://www.ama-assn.org/amednews/2013/01/14/bisa0114.htm (accessed February 14, 2013).

3. Catalyst for Payment Reform, Press Release, March 26, 2013, http://www.catalyze paymentreform.org/images/documents/release (accessed March 28, 2013).

4. Marcia James, "Successful Partnerships in Practice: A Payer Perspective," *MGMA Connexion*, 13, no.4 (2013): 38–40.

5. Wayne J. Guglielmo, "This Doctor Made P4P Work – You Can Too." *Medical Economics*, 85, no.14 (2008): 34-6, 42-4.

6. Craig Pederson and Theodore Praxel, MD, "Leveraging Marshfield Clinic's Practice Demonstration Experience in a 'Value-Based' Environment" (presentation at MGMA Annual Conference, October 23–26, 2011).

7. Charles Fiegl, "Medicare Pay: Insurers Preview a Post-SGR World," *amednews* (February 4, 2013), http://www.ama-assn.org/amednews/2013/02/04/gvsa0204.htm (accessed February 14, 2013).

8. *Medicare Physician Payment: Private-Sector Initiatives Can Help Inform CMS Quality and Efficiency Incentive Efforts*, GAO-13-160 (Government Accountability Office, December 2012), www.gao.gov/assets/660/651102.pdf.

9. *Theory and Reality of Value-Based Purchasing: Lessons from the Pioneers*. AHCPR Publication No. 98-0004 (Rockville, MD: Agency for Health Care Policy and Research, November 1997), http://www.ahrq.gov/qual/meyerrpt.htm (accessed February 25, 2013).

10. "Meaningful Use EHR Incentive Payments Near $13 Billion," *MGMA Washington Connexion*, April 17, 2013.

11. MGMA Government Affairs Staff, "Final 2013 Medicare Physician Fee Schedule Lays Groundwork for Value-Based Payment Modifier," *Washington Link*, January 2013, 20–22, http://www.mgma.com/workarea/downloadasset.aspx?id=1373088 (accessed January 24, 2013).

12. Mark W. Stanton, "Expanding Patient-Centered Care to Empower Patients and Assist Providers," *Research in Action*, Agency for Healthcare Research and Quality, Issue 5, 2002, http://www.ahrq.gov/research/findings/factsheets/patient-centered/ria-issue5/ (accessed March 1, 2013).

13. *MGMA Patient-Centered Care: 2012 Status and Prospects Report* (Englewood, CO: MGMA-ACMPE, 2012).

14. Mary Mourar, *Experts Answer 95 New Practice Management Questions* (Englewood, CO: Medical Group Management Association: 2012), 256.

15. NCQA, "PCMH & CPSP Eligibility," http://www.ncqa.org/Programs/Recognition/PatientCenteredMedicalHomePCMH/BeforeLearnItPCMHEligibility.aspx (accessed February 25, 2013).

16. NCQA Standards Workshop, Patient-Centered Medical Home, PCMH 2011, http://www.ncqa.org/Portals/0/Programs/Recognition/RPtraining/PCMH%202011%20standards%201-3%20%20workshop_2.3.12.pdf (accessed April 5, 2013).

17. MGMA Government Affairs, "CMMI Announces Payers in Comprehensive Primary Care Initiative," *MGMA Washington Connexion*, June 20, 2012, http://www.mgma.com/article.aspx?id=1371229 (accessed February 25, 2013).

18. R.S. Raskas L.M. Latts, J.R. Hummel, D. Wenners, H. Levine, and S.R. Nussbaum, "Early Results Show WellPoint's Patient-Centered Medical Home Pilots Have Met Some Goals for Costs, Utilization, and Quality," *Health Affairs*, 31, no.9 (2012): 2002–2009.

19. Emily Berry, "What's Behind WellPoint's Pay Raise for Primary Care Doctors?" *amednews* (February 13, 2012), http://www.ama-assn.org/amednews/2012/02/13/bisb0213.htm (accessed February 15, 2013).

20. Bruce Nash, MD, "Rewarding Primary Care Practice Reform with Physician Payment Reform: A Medical Home's Experience," *Guide to Physician Performance-Based Reimbursement: Payoffs from Incentives, Clinical Integration & Data Sharing* (Sea Girt, NJ: The Healthcare Intelligence Network, 2011), 22–31.

21. Charles Fiegl, "Medicare Pay: Insurers Preview a Post-SGR World," *amednews* (February 4, 2013), http://www.ama-assn.org/amednews/2013/02/04/gvsa0204.htm (accessed February 14, 2013).

22. Emily Berry, "Private Shared-Savings Deal Puts Half of Future Raises at Hospital System at Risk," *amednews* (July 31, 2012), http://www.ama-assn.org/amednews/2012/07/30/bisd0731.htm (accessed February 14, 2013).

23. See note 21 above.

24. See note 22 above.

25. David N. Gans, "You Don't Know What You Don't Know: Information Needs for Future Payment Systems" (presentation at MGMA Financial Management and Payer Contracting Conference, Phoenix, AZ, February 25, 2013).

26. Ibid.

27. Miranda Franco, "Evaluating Medicare ACOs and Bundled Payment Initiatives," *MGMA Connexion* (January 2013), 35–36.

28. "UnitedHealthcare Introduces New Cancer Care Payment Model," *Managed Care Outlook*, 23, no.24, (2010): 10–11.

29. See note 25 above.

30. Debra Bokur, "Can Global Payment Improve on Fee for Service and Capitation and Lower Healthcare Costs?" *MGMA Connexion* supplement, "How to Get Paid" (May/June 2012), http://www.mgma.com/workarea/mgma_downloadasset.aspx?id=1370833 (accessed March 2, 2013).

31. Robert Mechanic, Palmira Santos, Bruce Landon, and Michael Chernew, "Medical Group Responses to Global Payment: Early Lessons from the 'Alternative Quality Contract' in Massachusetts," *Health Affairs*, 30, no.9 (2011): 1734–1742.

32. See note 25 above.

33. Robert Mechanic and Darren E. Zinner, "Many Large Medical Groups Will Need to Acquire New Skills and Tools to Be Ready for Payment Reform," *Health Affairs*, 31, no.9 (2012): 1984–1992.

34. National Quality Forum, Community Tool to Align Measurement, http://www.qualityforum.org/AlignmentTool/ (accessed September 4, 2013).

35. Justin Chamblee, CPA, "Future Concepts in Physician Compensation" (presentation at MGMA Financial Management and Payer Contracting Conference, Phoenix, AZ, February 25, 2013).

36. William B. Weeks, Stephen S. Rauh, Eric B. Wadsworth, and James N. Weinstein, "The Unintended Consequences of Bundled Payments," *Annals of Internal Medicine*, 158, no.1 (2013): 62–64.

CHAPTER 5

Special Issues in Physician Compensation

Different issues that impact physician compensation methodology will develop in the life of a medical practice and in the lives of the physicians within it which will have to be addressed. Different stages in physicians' careers and personal lives impact their goals and behaviors. Practice mergers and growth create stress between specialties and departments, especially in multispecialty practices. Other issues relate to time devoted to practice functions, such as administrative or marketing activities, and whether physicians should be compensated for these endeavors. When these challenges develop, the practice must decide whether the issues can be handled on a case-by-case basis, with performance evaluations, or if changes in the compensation methodology are required.

The current issues and questions in the practice should have been identified during Step 3 (collect data) of the Decision Pathways physician compensation development process (discussed in chapter 2). Physician input during this step should identify any concerns or future plans that could impact compensation distribution. The issues and questions that could currently impact the practice or arise in the future include:

- What if a physician wants to change to a part-time schedule?

- Should a physician we're hiring be on the same compensation formula as the rest of us?

- What do we do if a physician doesn't want to buy into the practice?

- What if someone wants to stop being on call?

- How do we handle the stress developed from becoming a large multispecialty practice?

- Should revenue from nonphysician providers (NPPs) be included in the compensation pool, and if so, how should it be distributed?

- How do we distribute revenue from ancillary services?

- Should the managing partner and the executive committee be compensated for their time?

- Should we include nonclinical activities that support the group's mission?

- How do we address physician income earned outside of the practice?

Some issues can be handled with adjustments within the practice, but others can be more difficult or disruptive to address and require modifications within the compensation plan. When the compensation committee is conducting interviews with physicians, it should ask about these issues. Does the current compensation plan handle these issues adequately? If not, why not and how should they be handled? Are there potential issues that should be addressed now before they affect physician satisfaction or retention? The review of the practice documents and organizational mission, goals, and strategic plan, conducted during the information-gathering step, will also bring to light any issues that should be addressed.

Physicians' Career Stages

Physicians, like others, pass through different stages in their careers that will result in changes in knowledge, skill, work effort, and goals. Compensation plans that are flexible and adjust to these stages will contribute to maintaining physician satisfaction and a more congenial work environment. The main career stages and their related factors include:

- New physician
  - First year
  - Practice ownership and buy-in
- Mid career
- Late career
  - Transition to retirement

New Physicians

First-Year Physicians

Physicians recruited out of residency will be young and enthusiastic but new to the community, the practice, and the profession. They cannot be expected to perform at the productivity level of experienced physicians in the practice. They will perform best if supported for the first one to three years and mentored by other practice physicians. This time period will also enable them to build a patient panel and referral base. Productivity may be accelerated when the new physician is inheriting a depart-ing physician's practice.

Accommodating starting physicians will depend on the compensation methodol-ogy for the practice. A popular compensation formula for starting physicians is the straight salary. A guaranteed salary will provide an actual figure to attract physicians during the negotiation step of the recruitment process. The guaranteed salary will also provide a steady income for the physician during the process of learning and building patient capacity.

If straight salary is the compensation base of the other practice physicians, then there is less of an issue. If the medical practice uses a productivity-based methodology, the physician should be started on a salary and then transitioned to the productivity plan over a period of time.

How quickly the transition to the productivity-based plan can occur will depend on several factors:

- Is the new physician building a practice from scratch or inheriting an estab-lished practice from a retiring physician?

- Does he or she have an opportunity to build patient volume through educa-tion programs and/or marketing to referral sources?

- Is there enough patient demand to quickly build the physician's patient panel?

- Is there adequate support in the practice to mentor the physician and provide the needed nursing and other staff?

- Are established practice physicians willing to divert some of their patients to the new physician?

The practice administrator needs to evaluate each situation to determine a reasonable incentive plan that encourages productivity with attainable benchmarks over time. For example, the compensation plan could start with a guaranteed salary in the first year and then evolve to a lower guarantee with production incentives in the second year but without any downside risk. The full transition to a productivity-based for-mula would occur in the third year.

Determining the specific salary level will require evaluating the current market-place, the demand for the specialty of the new physician, and the results of a benchmarking analysis (described in chapter 2). Several salary surveys are available that can provide data on physician compensation for new or starting physicians (Exhibit 5.1). The guaranteed salary must also relate to what the physician will be able to make based on the predictions for patient panel size and productivity and expected compensation under a productivity-based compensation methodology.

EXHIBIT 5.1 ■ Resources for Starting-Physician Salary Data

MGMA Resources Available at www.mgma.com:
- The MGMA Physician Placement and Starting Salary Survey annually surveys medical practices to report compensation offered to first-year physicians, their benefits, and whether or not signing bonuses were offered.
- The MGMA Physician Compensation and Production Survey includes compensation and production data for physicians with one to two years of experience. Production numbers include collections, charges, and ambulatory encounters.

Additional Resources:
- American Medical Group Association, www.amga.org
- Sullivan Cotter Associates, www.sullivancotter.com/
- Merritt Hawkins *Review of Physician Recruiting Incentives*, www.merritthawkins.com

The physician will be disenchanted if the productivity-based compensation plan cannot sustain the initial salary.

The physician may also expect a signing bonus or assistance in paying off student loans or relocation costs. These will need to be considered as part of the recruitment package and in addition to the initial compensation for professional services. Sometimes increases in the recruiting incentives can offset lower-than-requested starting compensation.

The second-year transition to the full compensation plan can include productivity expectations or incentives for achieving or exceeding productivity targets. This will ease the physician onto a plan where compensation will be increasingly based on his or her own work efforts. The productivity targets should be based on the physician's performance the first year as well as benchmarks from the surveys. If the physician is performing below initial expectations, the benchmarks should be reviewed during discussion with the physician about his or her performance.

For example, the *MGMA Physician Compensation and Production Survey: 2012 Report Based on 2011 Data* indicates that the median number of ambulatory encounters for a family practitioner without obstetrics with one to two years of experience is approximately 3,000. This increases to 3,600 in the three- to seven-year range and approximately 3,800 by the eighth year of experience. This data implies that a new physician's productivity in this specialty is 79 percent of an experienced physician's productivity. The ratio was 74 percent when looking at collections. Meanwhile physicians with one to two years of experience earned approximately 83 percent of what physicians with eight or more years of experience earn. This may reflect the increasing demand for primary care physicians (PCPs).[1]

This brings up the concern that new physicians could earn more than experienced practice physicians if salary and productivity bonuses are set too high. While determining salary, it is necessary to consider current physician total compensation to ensure that compensation equity maintains a sense of fairness.

The transition plan should also include how nonproductivity measures will be integrated, including any incentives for patient satisfaction, quality, and outcome measures. In the second year, physicians can be presented with their first-year scores on these measures using a scorecard or performance report. However, it is better to delay including these measures in compensation until after the first year.

Newly Recruited, Experienced Physicians. New physicians are not necessarily recruited straight out of residency. They may be experienced physicians who are changing locations or medical practices. The transition to productivity-based plans for experienced physicians can occur at a different schedule than for young physicians. The pace of transition will depend on whether or not the physician is from outside of the community or from within the community and already has a patient and referral base that will be transferred to the new practice. Experienced physicians will expect compensation to be commensurate with their experience and previous compensation, making benchmarking and negotiation a more delicate process.

Two-Physician Families. An additional issue in physician recruitment is when a spouse is also a physician. The practice may be looking for one physician in a specific specialty, but that physician won't sign up unless a position is offered to the spouse that the practice may or may not need. Another issue is when the spouses are in the same specialty and they want to share a practice – two part-time physicians putting in the hours of one full-time equivalent (FTE). The two physicians may be in different specialties but only want to work part time and live on the combined income. Logistically, this may or may not work in the practice.

Another issue is when a physician and his or her spouse are hired, and one of them becomes dissatisfied with the practice. If one wants to leave, then the group may end up losing both. These situations make it tricky to offer compensation arrangements and work schedules that will keep both physicians happy. Dealing with the two-physician family isn't impossible; basically, you are dealing with two part-time physicians that should be addressed the same way other part-time positions are addressed. It may take some extra effort and care to address the objectives of both the physicians and the practice, including developing an exit strategy if the situation does not work out.

Practice Ownership and Buy-in

In physician-owned medical practices, the transition of a new physician from a guaranteed salary to a full compensation plan usually will match the transition from an employee to a shareholder or owner of the group practice. New physicians on a guaranteed salary for the first one to two years will frequently become eligible for buy-in at the third year. Some practices have an operating entity that employs all physicians and a separate entity that owns the equipment and real estate. Typically, only owners in the operating entity will be allowed to buy into the second entity. Ownership provides the opportunity to receive distribution of profits, including from ancillary services, which are distributed among all shareholders. The formula for profit distribution will vary depending on percentage of ownership of each physician and the corporate structure of the practice with its related tax code and other regulatory requirements. See chapter 6 for more information on the legal and regulatory requirements.

In recent years, there has been an increase in physicians who are hesitant to buy into practices. This may be due to concerns about how long they will want to stay with the same practice and location, as well as the cost of buying in compared with the benefits. The idea of the value of medical practices has been changing as the goodwill value is no longer respected as much as it was. Many physicians also think of the medical practice as a workplace rather than an equity and retirement investment as the previous generations did.

If practice ownership is not desired by recently recruited physicians, the practice should consider options to recognize the difference between owners and nonowners. Shareholders carry the risk and expense of becoming an owner and deserve recognition within the compensation structure. Shareholders may receive distribution of profits, including from ancillary services or different facilities owned by the group, that nonowners don't receive. This distribution must comply with the Stark law (see chapter 6). Another option is to increase compensation for owners by 5 to 10 percent above nonowners. This can be handled with a separate compensation pool or by adding a bonus to owners' compensation.

Some medical groups, especially very large practices, limit ownership to a few physicians and only allow physicians who have many years with the practice to become shareholders. In these practices, employed physicians are compensated via a different formula, frequently a salary or salary plus incentive.

Mid-Career Physicians

Physicians in the mid-career stage are at their greatest productivity and compensation, especially between 8 and 17 years of experience. They should be participating fully in the group's compensation formula. As long as the compensation methodology is reviewed every one to three years to address internal and external issues that arise, the physicians at this stage should continue to maximize their contribution to the practice and its goals. The main compensation-related issues that may occur during this stage are the requests for a part-time schedule or changes in call coverage. Physicians at this stage will also be expected to participate in practice leadership.

Late-Career Physicians

Physicians who have worked many productive years and are approaching retirement frequently want to continue working but on a reduced schedule. These physicians will usually want to reduce or stop taking call and go to a part-time schedule. Each practice will need to discuss whether or not to allow this change and how to handle the transition toward retirement. Decisions include how much reduction in call and hours to allow, how to handle compensation, and if the physician must have been with the practice a minimum number of years to be eligible. Groups may choose to set a time limit – two to three years, for example – on how long a physician can serve a reduced schedule prior to retiring.

If the request for a part-time schedule is granted, the compensation and expense allocation can be adjusted as described in the following sections. Some practices will shift a transitioning physician off of the main compensation formula to a straight salary, thereby reducing the amount the physician may receive from profit sharing or other revenue.

Call Schedules and Compensation

The two types of call coverage are group practice call coverage and being available for emergencies in hospitals as may be required by hospital by-laws. Both types may need to be addressed in medical practices. Increasingly, physicians are receiving stipends from hospitals to support their emergency services. This is especially true with certain specialties. Compensation for hospital call coverage can be handled in the same manner as other outside revenue, discussed later in this section.

Obligations to cover call for the group practice are handled differently depending on the specialty, practice, and setting. In some situations, there may not be an adequate number of specialists within the group to cover call, and arrangements may be made to compensate NPPs or outside physicians to share the call requirements. For many groups, call coverage is expected of every physician and therefore is not compensated separately (Exhibit 5.2). However, during the life of a practice, situations may arise in which physicians are not able to participate in the call schedule or wish to cut back the amount of call.

Several options are available for handling compensation and changes in call coverage, as discussed in the following paragraphs.

EXHIBIT 5.2 ■ Call Coverage Type of Compensation Method Used

Compensation Type	Respondents/Providers	Percentage
No additional compensation	1,184	29.97
Daily stipend	1,429	36.18
Annual stipend	487	12.33
Per shift	325	8.23
Hourly rate	279	7.06
Monthly stipend	134	3.39
Weekly stipend	26	0.66
Per wRVU	18	0.46

Source: *MGMA Medical Directorship and On-Call Compensation Survey: 2013 Report Based on 2012 Data*, Englewood, CO: Medical Group Management Association, 2013.

Determine a dollar amount per call shift. This amount can then be subtracted from the compensation of the physician who is giving up the call and applied to those who increase their call. The practice can serve as a broker to track the call schedule changes and compensation. Another option is to have one physician negotiate directly with another physician, and they handle the transfer of money without administrator involvement. This method can be applied for an occasional call change (e.g., when a physician needs to attend a child's evening program) as well as for long-term changes.

Different dollar amounts are usually applied to evening weekday call and weekend call (from Friday evening to early Monday morning). Groups can arrive at the actual dollar amount by asking physicians how much they are willing to pay to have another physician take their call and how much they would want to receive for taking call. The average of the two may be acceptable to most physicians. These amounts can also be benchmarked with the *MGMA Medical Directorship and On-Call Compensation Survey* report that tracks compensation or stipend amounts broken out by the type of call coverage, facility, and location.

Reduce the physician's total compensation to reflect the reduction in call. This method is better for long-term periods of reduction in call. The reduction can be done by a percentage, frequently in the 15–35 percent range, or by a set dollar amount ($25,000, for example). The actual amount will have to be negotiated based on what other physicians in the practice believe is fair depending on the additional burden it puts on them.

Apply an RVU amount per call shift or hours of call. Compensation can then be adjusted using the compensation per RVU (relative value unit) ratio. This option works well in practices with RVU-based compensation methodology. For example, a practice can apply a value of three or four Current Procedural Terminology® (CPT®)

EXHIBIT 5.3 ■ Method Used to Accommodate Part-Time Physicians

	Better Performing Practices	Other Practices
Paid less and provided fewer benefits	44.83%	35.83%
Changed the overhead rate	16.26%	9.84%
Encouraged job sharing rather than part-time employment	5.42%	6.69%
Part-time physicians were not employed at the practice	27.59%	29.13%
Other accommodations for part-time physicians	10.78%	8.66%

Source: *MGMA Performance and Practices of Successful Medical Groups: 2012 Report Based on 2011 Data.* Englewood, CO: Medical Group Management Association, 2012.

99213* office visits per hour of call and determine the number of hours per call shift. These RVU values are added to the total to determine the physician's total compensation for the pay period.

Part-Time Physicians

There are many reasons that physicians may request part-time status, including:

- Taking care of children;
- Taking care of an aging parent;
- Difficulty of managing a household on a full-time schedule; or
- Transitioning toward retirement.

The number of part-time physicians has steadily increased. Almost 10 percent of physicians responding to the MGMA Physician Compensation and Production Survey worked less than a full-time schedule in 2012.[2] As many as 25 percent of physicians in large medical groups worked a part-time schedule in 2011, compared with 13 percent in 2005, according to one survey. That survey also shows that many male physicians are asking for part-time status: 22 percent in the 2011 survey compared with 44 percent for women.[3]

Medical practices can use different solutions to address the question when a physician requests part-time status, as shown in Exhibit 5.3. Reduction in compensation and benefits was the most frequent response provided by responding medical practices. Physicians on straight salary or salary plus bonus can receive a reduced salary

---

* CPT © 2014 American Medical Association. All rights reserved.

prorated to the reduction in hours worked. For example, if a physician moves to three-quarters of a full-time schedule, then the salary is reduced to 75 percent of his or her previous salary. A similar reduction can occur for physicians on equal share. Productivity-based physicians will see a reduction in productivity with a reduction in hours. Their compensation will be reduced automatically based on the change in their productivity measure.

Expense allocation may be more difficult to determine than compensation. If full-time employees are still needed to support the physician, along with a dedicated office, the fixed and indirect expenses do not decrease as much as the revenue and compensation will decrease. For this reason, it may make sense to allocate expenses at the same rate for part-time physicians as for full-timers. If physicians object to receiving full expense allocation, it may be necessary to compromise and lower the amount allocated. Options for determining expense allocation include basing it on the percentage of FTE hours worked or calculating the ratio of collections or RVUs generated by the physician compared with FTE physicians (as discussed in chapter 3). All direct expenses (including insurance, continuing medical education, benefits) can be allocated to the part-time physician, and indirect and variable expenses distributed based on percentage of patients seen, hours worked, or their percentage of total collections or work relative value units (wRVUs). Another option is for the practice to absorb overhead costs for part-time physicians but reduce the compensation for the physician to make up the difference.

Job Sharing

An alternative for handling part-time requests is to find an NPP or another physician to fill in the gap. Job sharing will let two physicians or a physician and an NPP work part-time schedules but maintain practice revenues. If it is true job sharing, including sharing an office, expenses will equal that of one FTE. However, if two offices are required or the compensation and benefits aren't evenly split, expense and compensation calculations can be complicated.

Compensation and expense allocation can be based on either of the options presented above for both providers. If expenses are allocated to each physician, then the job sharing providers can split the indirect cost allocation based on their relative percentages of time worked (50-50 percent or 60-40 percent) and assume their direct costs.

Nonphysician Providers' Supervision and Revenue Distribution

The presence of NPPs has increased over the years for several reasons. NPPs can handle more routine visits leaving physicians free to handle more procedures and complex

EXHIBIT 5.4 ■ FTE Nonphysician Providers per Responding Group Practice

Number of NPPs	Multispecialty Practices	Primary Care Practices
1 FTE or fewer	15.00%	26.80%
2 to 3 FTEs	12.33%	35.05%
4 to 6 FTEs	15.00%	21.65%
7 FTEs or more	57.67%	16.49%

Source: *MGMA Cost Survey for Primary Care Practices* and *MGMA Cost Survey for Multispecialty Practices: 2012 Reports Based on 2011 Data*. Englewood, CO: Medical Group Management Association, 2012.

visits. They also increase patient access when there isn't enough demand to hire a full-time physician or where there is a physician shortage. Now many group practices employ several NPPs (Exhibit 5.4).

Depending on state regulations, physicians may be required to provide close supervision overseeing the NPPs and reviewing their recommendations, prescriptions, and so forth. Regulations may only require that the physician be present for a consult, if needed. If close supervision is required, the time spent may impact a physician's productivity and, therefore, compensation if based on productivity.

The compensation plan will have to address the issues of time spent supervising NPPs and distribution of revenue generated by the NPPs. Practice settings will determine how these issues are handled. If one or more NPPs were hired by one physician to work directly with him or her, that physician may be assuming all the risk for the time, costs, and malpractice concerns of the NPP and therefore may deserve to be allocated all of the revenue generated by that provider. In this case, the NPP's salary, benefits, and other expenses are directly allocated to that physician. This situation can lead to increased stress within a practice if other physicians believe the situation is unfair or inhibiting the physician from supporting a decision to recruit another physician.

A better option is for the practice to assume the hiring, compensation, and revenue sharing of all NPPs within the practice. In this option, NPP revenue is added to the total revenue of the practice rather than to the supervising physician and distributed as part of the total compensation methodology. Supervising physicians can be compensated with an hourly rate or stipend paid per week or month. To determine the amount, ask the physicians to think about the average time spent supervising in a day or week, usually only a few minutes at a time. Ask physicians what would be a reasonable compensation for that time. Networking with peers can also be used to arrive at estimates for NPP supervision stipends.

Large Group Practice Challenges

As described in chapter 1, group practice size has increased over the years as solo and small practices find it difficult to compete in today's marketplace and to handle the regulatory and information technology demands. The growth of practices has increased their complexity and the challenges of developing compensation formulas that satisfy all the physicians in a practice (or at least leave them equally unsatisfied). This is especially true if practice mergers combine physicians from previous practices and cultures. These challenges will need to be included during the compensation development process or they will be addressed under stressful conditions later.

With an increase in the number of physicians, odds are that one or more of the issues discussed throughout this chapter will arise. However, some issues will be unique because of the size of the practice, especially if the group has more than one specialty. Differences in reimbursement, work effort, procedure versus office visit emphasis, and so on, will strain the relationships of the physicians who may target the compensation formula as the blame. This increases the need to include a variety of physicians in the compensation plan review and development process.

Multispecialty practices with a mix of PCPs and specialists will contend with the widespread differences in specialty reimbursement and work styles putting additional strain on compensation systems. PCPs may be jealous of the increased compensation of the specialists, and specialists may believe they are subsidizing the PCPs. These differences can be exaggerated with revenue from ancillary services offered by the specialists. However, specialists should realize that much of their income is from referrals from the PCPs. Emphasis should be placed on the group's mission and culture over these differences, but there are measures that can be taken in revenue and expense allocation to minimize the potential conflict.

One solution is to separate revenue and expenses by department so each specialty or department acts more as an independent practice. Some of the revenue would be kept by the group to cover overhead and shared activities. Any allocations regarding ancillary services revenue and expenses must be considered in light of the Stark law (see chapter 6). The practice may use one compensation formula for all physicians or use different formulas, especially between PCPs and specialists. It is still necessary to recruit and retain physicians, so the ultimate test of a complex formula is how close compensation comes to appropriate benchmarks.

Merging practices into a larger group raises the difficult question of how to handle compensation formulas. A few groups have chosen to keep the previous compensation formulas rather than trying to develop a new, integrated method. This may work for some groups but will prevent others from ever truly bonding as one group practice with a shared culture. Leaders from the merging groups or a committee with representatives from all groups should meet and develop a compensation formula that instills a sense of unity, common goals, and effort. If physicians can't agree on a mutually acceptable model, some newly merged practices will retain their original compensation plan for a year or two and then work to transition into a common methodology.

Practice Leadership and Citizenship

As practices grow in size, administering them becomes more complex. Leadership demands more time, and more committees are formed to deal with a variety of issues. One of the internal challenges is how to encourage and recognize physicians for serving in practice leadership roles.

Managing Partners and Medical Directors

Historically, physicians may have rotated as managing partners or medical directors in practices, and the amount of hours to serve in these roles was minimal. Physicians were expected to serve on their rotation and with minimal interruption to clinical activities, so no additional compensation was offered. As practices grew in size, the amount of time increased and physicians volunteered or were elected to serve in leadership roles rather than serving on a rotation. Practices also found that the rotation methodology is subject to the various levels of the current incumbent's skills. With the increased demand on physician leaders' time, their productivity and compensation were impacted. Groups had to decide whether practice leadership activities are expected and included within the compensation methodology or if compensation should be offered separately. Without additional compensation, groups may find it increasingly difficult to get physicians to volunteer or accept the leadership positions, even for those physicians who find themselves suited to management and leadership roles. This is especially a problem where compensation is based on clinical production and the leaders are expected to sacrifice productivity and/or personal time to fulfill leadership activities.

When compensation is offered for managing partners or directors, there are several ways to offer it. Responses to the MGMA Medical Directorship and On-Call Compensation Survey show that the most frequent methods are hourly rate, annual stipend, and monthly stipend (Exhibit 5.5). This MGMA survey also provides benchmark figures for compensation rates for medical directors and their responsibilities. The actual amount of the stipend will depend on the specialty, number and importance of responsibilities, amount of time spent in the responsibilities, and what physicians agree to. If leadership responsibilities reduce clinical time substantially, the practice may consider the physician to be a part-time clinical physician and base their compensation and expense allocation accordingly, and then provide enough stipend to raise the total compensation to the approximate level of a full-time clinician. These compensation methods can also be applied to other leadership positions, including board positions and department heads that demand substantial time.

EXHIBIT 5.5 ■ Type of Compensation Method for a Medical Director

Method	Number of Respondents	Percentage
Hourly rate	585	41.17
Monthly stipend	405	28.50
Annual stipend	347	24.42
Deferred compensation	4	0.28
Weekly stipend	1	0.07
Other method	52	3.66
No additional compensation	27	1.90

Source: *MGMA Medical Directorship and On-Call Compensation Survey: 2013 Report Based on 2012 Data.* Englewood, CO: Medical Group Management Association, 2013.

In determining stipends or total compensation for medical directors and other physician leaders, groups can consider whether incentives should be included to better align the physicians' behavior with organizational goals and performance. Leadership incentives can incorporate similar goals and incentives for other physicians in the group or goals limited to their performance. Ideally, physicians holding these positions should also have a job description and frequent evaluations of their leadership functions.

Along with organizational financial and quality goals, leadership incentives can include factors such as:

- The ability to execute strategy;
- Recruitment and retention of physicians;
- Professional growth and development of physicians; and
- Achieving organizational long-term, growth, quality, or enterprise goals.[4]

Similar questions regarding physician incentive formulas can be applied to physician leadership incentives:

- What percentage of the compensation should be based on incentives?
- What incentives should be included and how will they be measured?
- Will the measures be based on individual or organizational performance, or a combination?
- Which leaders will be included in the incentive system?

Committee and Citizenship Activities

Participation in practice administration and leadership includes time spent on committees such as compensation, executive, financial, quality, and others. Committee participation is usually less demanding than leadership roles, thus compensation may be handled differently. Groups may also want to encourage and recognize time spent to develop new service lines, promote the practice in the community, proctor new medical students, develop patient education materials, and endorse similar activities that support the organizational goals and promotion.

If groups expect every physician to participate on committees or in other activities, then no additional compensation may be offered, although it may be a factor in physician performance evaluations. Other groups may choose to add recognition and reward to invite and increase participation. If physicians are asked to support a specific project with defined objectives, the incentive or reward can be a one-time bonus.

Practice citizenship is often included in incentive compensation, as described later in several examples in chapter 10. One example is the service recognition program developed by one primary care practice. A point system was developed to recognize committee involvement and other practice citizenship activities. Physicians were awarded one point for each committee they participated in, as long as they attended at least 50 percent of the meetings. Distribution from an incentive pool was made at year end, depending on the total number of points.[5]

Ancillary Services and Designated Health Services Revenue

As discussed in chapter 6 on legal and regulatory issues, the Stark law limits how revenue from designated health services is distributed to physicians. The law was passed to limit physicians' financial benefit from referring to services in which they owned a financial stake and received a share of the profits. The law provides specific recommendations on how DHS (designated health services) revenue can be distributed to physicians under the group practice exemption. See chapter 6 for more information.

Outside Revenue

Physicians often serve in roles outside of the practice for which they receive reimbursement. Examples of outside activities include:

- Hospital call coverage;
- Medical directorships at hospitals, nursing homes, ambulatory surgery centers, and other healthcare facilities;

- Honorariums for speaking or publishing;

- Principal investigator responsibilities for clinical trials;

- Providing expert testimony; and

- Providing medical services at sporting events.

How the group handles compensation for these services will depend on the physicians' employment agreements, practice by-laws, contract to provide the services (is the contract with the practice or individual physician?), and how much time is spent away from practice activities. The practice culture should be reflected in these documents and passed through into the compensation methodology. Groups may expect the practice to receive the income and pass it through to the physician, either as part of the total practice compensation pool or directly to the physician. A percentage of the payment will frequently be retained by the practice to help cover the overhead costs and any lost revenue from the physician's time away from the practice. In other groups, physicians may keep all outside revenue, especially if it has minimal effect on clinical time. Reimbursement for activities that occur on a physician's own time and are not connected with the group, such as covering sporting events, may be retained by the physician.[6]

Community Participation

Some physicians may have strong beliefs about promoting community health and volunteering in community health events and services. Medical groups may also promote community involvement as part of their mission and as a means to promote and market the practice. Examples of such events and activities include community education presentations, not-for-profit health screenings, volunteering at free clinics, proctoring medical students, and conducting physical exams for sport leagues. Including these activities within a compensation plan will depend on whether or not community participation is expected as part of the organization's mission and whether the organization wants to recognize and reward the time and effort. For some practices with a strong orientation toward community service, participation is a factor in physicians' performance reviews and may be included as part of incentive bonuses.

For example, one primary care practice believed community service was important enough that service recognition was compensated by a tax-and-value scale. Group physicians contributed to a fund with a $1,000 "tax" per physician per year. In such a system, each activity is assigned a value, such as 1.57 points for community presentations, 2 points for peer presentations, and 1.71 points for nursing home visits. Caps are applied to develop a maximum number of points for certain activities. All the points are tallied at the end of the year, and each physician receives a portion of the community service fund based on his or her tally.[7]

Behavioral Incentives and Subjective Measures

As mentioned in chapter 1, one of the internal challenges that may require changes to the compensation plan is behavioral issues. If a lack of desired behavior is impacting practice financial or strategic success, incentives or penalties may be needed to change the behavior. The practice leadership and compensation committee must decide if the issue is related to one physician or is systemic. If it is one physician, the medical director should address the issue with the provider. If the problem is more systemic, then the compensation plan can include incentives to try to correct the issue.

Using stipends or other compensation and incentives to encourage participation in practice administration and committees has already been discussed. Other issues that may arise include:

- Failure to complete medical records and charges;
- Hesitancy to use electronic health records, e-prescribing, or other information technology tools;
- Lack of team participation; and
- Relations with nurses or other employees.

Including behavior incentives in compensation formulas can be handled similar to the quality and satisfaction metrics discussed in chapter 4. The factors should be measurable by objective means as much as possible; for example, completion of 90 percent of charges within three days or 85 percent of prescriptions handled through the e-prescribing function.

Subjective measures are more difficult to manage and can result in "personality contests." Examples of subjective measures are peer rating systems and employee satisfaction surveys. If the survey tools are well developed, they can serve a useful function; but since they are subjective, they should be handled differently than objective measurements. One option is to apply the subjective measures in comparison with average scores for all physicians. Determine the average or median score for each survey tool and rate physicians as above, at, or below average; physicians with higher-than-average ratings receive higher or additional bonuses. Physicians with below-average scores either receive no additional bonus or can even be penalized with a deduction in compensation. The latter option is usually not well received but may be required.

Trying to address individual behavior issues by tweaking the compensation formula may not work, and may even be counterproductive. Some issues should be addressed directly in a one-on-one manner with the problem physician.

Compensation Pool for Special Issues

Addressing the challenges and issues described in this chapter frequently involves providing physicians with additional compensation, which requires a source of funding. The value-based compensation incentives described in chapter 4 may be funded through incentive reimbursement payments from payers. There isn't an external source for funding internally developed incentive compensation. The group must decide whether funding will come from withholding compensation from physicians until goals (e.g., committee participation) are achieved or setting aside a portion of the total compensation pool. The latter is usually preferred since physicians will then view the additional compensation as a bonus. Withholds are usually seen in a more negative light.

Compensation for physician leadership can also be considered part of total practice expenses, deducted from net revenue. This is especially true for compensation for full-time or nearly full-time leaders with minimal, if any, clinical time.

The primary care practice described earlier in the "Community Participation" section developed a unique alternative of taxing their physicians each year to contribute to the incentive pool. This was agreed to by all physicians. Physicians who were too busy with young families appreciated the tax, knowing that it was their contribution to support the group effort.[8]

End Notes

1. Jeffrey B. Milburn, MBA, CMPE, "Ease New Physicians into Productivity-Based Compensation Plans," *MGMA e-Source* (November 9, 2010), http://mgma.com/article .aspx?id=39957 (accessed February 13, 2013).

2. *MGMA Physician Compensation and Production Survey: 2013 Report Based on 2012 Data* (Englewood, CO: Medical Group Management Association, 2013).

3. Robert Lowes, "1 in 4 Physicians Employed by Large Groups Are Part-Time," *Medscape Medical News* (March 21, 2012), http://www.cejkasearch.com/wp-content/uploads/ Medscape_03.21_-1-in-4-Physicians-Are-Part-Time.pdf (accessed March 12, 2013).

4. Mary Heymans, "Physician Leadership Incentive Compensation Plans," *Becker's Hospital Review* (June 14, 2011), http://www.beckershospitalreview.com/compensation-issues/ physician-leadership-incentive-compensation-plans.html (accessed April 22, 2013).

5. L. Rousche, "Giving, and Getting, Back to Your Practice and Community." *Medical Economics*, 88, no.11 (2011): 53–54.

6. Marshall Baker, "Physician Compensation – Addressing the Gray Areas," MGMA webinar, November 10, 2011.

7. See note 4 above.

8. Ibid.

CHAPTER 6

Legal and Regulatory Issues in Compensation Plan Development

Thomas Godar
Shareholder, Whyte Hirschboeck Dudek
Madison Office HR Practice Leader

and

Barbara Zabawa
Shareholder, Whyte Hirschboeck Dudek
Healthcare Practice Leader

Although many employment relationships do not have the benefit of a written agreement, nearly all relationships for physicians are confirmed through written employment contracts. While these contracts cover a variety of different issues, many of which are commonplace to all employment settings, often a significant focus is on compensation as a variable component. However, many other issues are also components of a well-crafted physician employment agreement.

Physician Employment Agreements

Forming the Contract

The initiation of negotiations over employment often relates to specific terms, such as compensation, practice support, specific descriptions of opportunities, and the like. The contractual relationship begins with exchanging general and then specific terms and conditions of employment. The contract is formed when one party makes an offer of employment to another, that offer is accepted, and consideration is exchanged or will be exchanged as a result of this relationship. Although there can be oral contracts, in almost all cases, these physician agreements should be reduced to writing and signed. Indeed, in many states, an oral contract purporting to last more than one year would be unenforceable under the doctrine of "Statute of Frauds." This written document, signed and dated, then becomes the centerpiece for the relationship.

Normally, the board of directors of a clinic has either delegated the responsibility to negotiate and enter physician agreements to the clinic president or executive director, or the clinic board of directors or executive board will take up any contract and authorize the clinic to move forward. Likewise, hospitals engaging in hiring practices have normally delegated this authority to certain hospital executives. Delegation of such authority with clear boundaries can aid in negotiations and hasten securing the services of a qualified candidate in this competitive arena. Of course, it is assumed the physician has the authority to enter into any agreement, but the initiation of employment is often contingent on such items as the state regulatory and licensing body approving the physician's application for practice privileges in the state, or hospitals or managed care organizations providing privileges or credentials, and further conditions of the physician's representation that he or she is not encumbered by any noncompetition or other obligations related to his or her last employment.

Once the contract is signed, the physician and the clinic or hospital should maintain an executed copy of the employment agreement in an easily accessible, though secure, place. Contracts that contain individual compensation or other personal information are routinely considered confidential, and, to the extent they are kept in some sort of electronic format, such versions should be password protected and accessible only on a need-to-know basis. It is suggested as well that if counsel worked with the employer in crafting the agreement or negotiating the final terms that counsel should also be provided with and maintain a final copy of the signed employment agreement.

Terms of the Agreement

As is emphasized throughout this book, any employment agreement ought to align with the goals and mission of the healthcare practice or hospital employer. Great care should be taken that the financial incentives line up with the practice's goals. A practice or hospital that is intent on emphasizing quality standards and a collegial workplace should be careful not to offer financial incentives that are driven exclusively by production and procedures. Further, if items such as collegiality are of high cultural value, the contract terms should reflect that and allow for termination if the physician is unable to provide care in such a collegial atmosphere. For instance, certain contracts might have a provision detailing what behaviors can constitute cause for termination, such as the following:

> *Physician's inability to practice collegially in the clinic setting or with Hospital staff, as determined by the Corporation, after written notice to Physician and a reasonable opportunity of not less than thirty (30) days to immediately and continually meet his obligation to practice in a collegial manner.*

The parties should also be careful lest a contract is laced with legalese or is written in terms that are ambiguous and left open to multiple interpretations for application. Indeed, courts may insist that if there are restrictions on postemployment activities, unclear language would either be construed against the employer or perhaps make the entire restrictive covenant unenforceable. Areas such as compensation practices, standards of care, and the like should be set forth in a way to allow both parties a clear understanding of the goals and expectations of the employment arrangement.

Termination Provisions

The most difficult part of an employment relationship is often the exit. If the contract is for a specific term, then there is one agreed-upon exit opportunity for both sides: the end of the contract term. However, physician agreements often have clauses that provide for an automatic renewal of the contract or opportunities for clinic ownership along with continued employment. However, not all relationships continue indefinitely. Although parties often anticipate a long employment relationship, nothing can be more difficult than either a quit or a termination, whether for cause or without cause, when the parties are fighting over patient access, information, deferred compensation, accounts receivable, bonuses, or payout of equity that was part of the relationship. To avoid these challenges, careful review of unlikely and unusual circumstances is necessary. For instance; the contract should answer the following questions:

- What constitutes cause to quit or be terminated, short of the contract term?
- If the physician received an advance as a recruitment incentive, need he or she pay that advance back upon early exit?
- Does repayment of an advance vary based on whether the physician voluntarily leaves or is forced out?
- If a recruitment incentive was provided to a physician by a hospital, is the physician responsible for repayment of any incentive that has not been waived or repaid? If so, how is payment achieved?
- May the physician walk down the street and open up a competing practice or work with a competing practice, even while receiving a stream of payments from receivables based on work performed while at the former clinic?
- How is repayment of equity calculated and when must it be paid to a departing physician/owner?
- What happens to compensation arrangements based on physician-related income to the practice when a physician leaves?
- What happens to equipment or other assets purchased by members of the group?

These questions should be answered with clarity while the parties are anticipating an excellent relationship, and not after the relationship has all but disintegrated.

Practice Tips

Along with the previously mentioned information, several ideas related to physician employment agreements that will protect the practice include the following:

- Treat substantial bonuses, moving allowance, and school loan payments as loans until an employee has worked for two or three years, during which the payments to or on behalf of the physician may be forgiven. However, be mindful of the tax implications and whether such bonuses are currently taxable, as income, or treated as a loan for tax purposes.

- Consider including an enforceable covenant not to compete, but with exceptions as necessary to promote continuity of patient care and adequate notice.

- Reduce or eliminate opportunities to receive a continuing stream of payments from accounts receivable if the physician is terminated for cause or leaves voluntarily without good reason.

- Identify the obligations, if any, of the parting physician to secure his or her own tail coverage when leaving the practice.

Typical Provisions in a Contract

The provisions in a contract, especially as they relate to compensation, can vary significantly, based on the drivers identified by the clinic or hospital. Often these compensation issues are addressed in an addendum to the agreement, so that the underlying terms and conditions may remain the same while the clinic changes the compensation provisions to suit the evolving practice or the maturing activities of a physician with the practice. If the compensation provision is subject to change, such flexibility should be set forth plainly in the agreement as well as repeated in any addendum. The clinic may wish to preserve the flexibility to reduce or reengineer the incentive formula or base compensation for a physician contract.

Sometimes examples of how a more complicated formula is applied may be an appropriate portion of any sort of compensation agreement. This may be particularly helpful when a practice has had a stable environment and the member physicians have become accustomed to an evolving compensation system, but the application of the system may not be apparent from the words used in the compensation provisions of the agreement or the compensation addendum. Specific examples of how the streams of clinic income or the expenses will be allocated to individual physicians or to the overall clinic can be helpful. Creating an example will also force a clinic administrator to think through the actual twists and turns of any particular compensation agreement.

The typical terms that may be found in an employment agreement for a physician are the term or length of time of an agreement; how either party might terminate the contract short of the term, or how the term may be extended, whether unilaterally or by mutual agreement; the corporation's duties, rights, and obligations, including its duty to bill and collect, manage, secure, and provide office and clinic facilities, equipment and supplies, and ancillary personnel, provide insurance, maintain and grant access to medical records, and provide compensation. Some agreements also include incentives to join a practice, such as a moving allowance, a recruitment bonus, payment of school loans, and the like. These items are sometimes identified as loans, forgiven after a period of time. However, the clinic or hospital must be aware that such "loans" may be characterized as compensation by taxing authorities.

The physician duties described in an employment agreement include definition of full- or part-time employment status; appropriate or inappropriate outside activities, retaining or providing to the clinic compensation for any outside activities; achieving and maintaining staff privileges at hospitals and ambulatory surgical centers; maintaining rights to bill services through Medicare/Medicaid or through the insurance with whom the clinic makes contracts; coverage requirements; cooperation in billing and collection; confidentiality and noncompetition agreements, if appropriate; and meeting professional standards while exercising independent professional judgment.

A termination section should include termination by the clinic for cause, with specific definitions, or for breach of the agreement; or by the physician for the clinic's breach of the agreement; or termination based on the physician's inability to perform the services outlined in the agreement.

Of course, contracts also contain "boilerplate" provisions such as provisions preventing the assignment of the agreement, adopting a particular state's governing law, prohibiting amendments or modification without writing, and so on.

Legal Cautions

Beyond the obvious advantage of having a clear and comprehensive agreement governing the compensation and relationship between a clinic and its physicians, whether those physicians are owners or employees, such employment agreements should conform to legal standards. Obviously, they should not be written in a way that discriminates against employees who are age 40 and older, which would violate the Age Discrimination Act and correlating state laws. Physicians who are able to competently practice should not be held to artificial standards demanding their retirement at a particular age. Likewise, physicians who suffer a disability – a mental or physical impairment that substantially limits major life activity – but are able to continue performing the primary functions of their position with or without reasonable accommodation should be allowed to continue contributing to the clinic in order to comply with the Americans with Disabilities Act of 1990 (ADA). Therefore, employment agreements that provide for automatic termination of employment because of a physician's absence due to disability for a set period of time may give rise to complaints under the ADA as not allowing an interactive process to play out in order to provide a reasonable accommodation to a disability. Under the ADA, a disability is generally defined as the inability of an otherwise qualified individual to perform the essential functions of the employment position, with or without reasonable accommodation.

Of course, there are also a myriad of tax issues that arise in any compensation scheme. A complete treatment of the implications of such issues is well beyond the scope of this book, but highlighting some of the most salient topics follows.

Taxation for a private clinic, not established as a not-for-profit corporation, will depend partially on whether the practice is organized as a corporation classified as a "C" corporation or as a corporation that has elected "subchapter S" designation for tax purposes. In traditional, physician-owned medical groups that are taxed as subchapter S corporations, partnership-like treatment of income will be applied as it is earned by the medical group. However, when a group practice is treated as a C corporation for tax purposes, the corporation pays taxes on earnings after compensation is deducted. To be deductible, such compensation must be reasonable. Amounts paid in excess of reasonable compensation would generally be treated as nondeductible dividends and not as compensation. In a subchapter S corporation, because of its flow-through treatment, the issue of paying more than reasonable compensation is generally not an issue. This may be an important distinction between the two types of taxation typically found in a privately owned clinic.

Compensation provided in hospital-owned or hospital-operated group practices or paid directly to physicians may be subject to other tests, including the Stark and anti-kickback laws, which are discussed in more detail below. Particularly if a hospital is a tax-exempt organization under section 501(c)(3) of the Internal Revenue Code (IRC), special requirements might apply. Under section 4958 of the IRC, compensation arrangements between the organization and the physician must support and promote the purpose of the tax-exempt organization, the amount of compensation actually paid is no more than "reasonable" compensation, and that the process of determining the compensation arrangements should be at arm's length and be determined by those other than the compensated physician or physician group. There should be caution about using the "net earnings" of a not-for-profit hospital as a measure of compensation. Such plans might consider capping incentive payments and making sure that such incentives are consistent with well-defined formulas related to the organization's charitable mission.

Further, the Internal Revenue Service (IRS) may also look carefully at loans from practices to either new or continuing physicians. Such loans carry imputed income of the interest if interest is not paid on a commercially reasonable basis. More problematic, "loans" may be characterized as current income, whether they be in the form of incentives to new employees or bonuses that may be subject to repayment, if these loans are routinely larger. For instance, in a recent decision regarding *The Vancouver Clinic, Inc., v. U.S., Inc.*, that was decided in April of 2013, the court found that forgivable loans paid to physicians at the time of the physician's recruitment and retention should have been treated as compensation with the accompanying withholding obligations. The court held that for such payments to be considered a loan, at least for tax purposes, there must be an unconditional promise to repay at the time the funds are advanced. This yields to a second consideration: whether the parties actually intend for the advance to be repaid at the time that it is made. If there is no intent of repayment, the transaction is not a loan. The court observed that the loans provided to the new physician would be forgiven by the clinic after five years of employment by the physician. The court found it was only in exceptional cases that anyone would actually repay the loan. Hence, the court considered these loans as compensation for services with all of the resulting obligations. Further, if a hospital "loans" a clinic or physician equipment, such as computers, or provides office facilities, the clinic should pay a commercially reasonable fee for such equipment or facilities.

It will be important to work with qualified financial and legal experts to make sure that any distributions or arrangements are properly accounted for as compensation, a loan, or payment of lease fees.

Stark Law

The Stark law seeks to deter an inclination to generate Medicare revenue through improper referrals by physicians. The Stark regulations are found at 42 CFR § 350, et seq., and implement section 1877 of the Social Security Act. The Stark law "generally prohibits a physician from making a referral under Medicare for designated health services to an entity with which the physician or a member of the physician's immediate family has a financial relationship."[1] As a result, the Stark law must have physician involvement in order to be implicated. There must also be a financial relationship, either through ownership or compensation, with an "entity" that provides "designated health services" (DHS) payable by the Medicare program.[2]

DHS includes 10 types of services, including:

1. Clinical laboratory services;

2. Physical therapy, occupational therapy, and outpatient speech-language pathology services;

3. Radiology and certain other imaging services;

4. Radiation therapy services and supplies;

5. Durable medical equipment and supplies;

6. Parenteral and enteral nutrients, equipment, and supplies;

7. Prosthetics, orthotics, and prosthetic devices and supplies;

8. Home health services;

9. Outpatient prescription drugs; and

10. Inpatient and outpatient hospital services.[3]

An "entity" includes a physician practice or hospital or other corporate entity that "furnishes" DHS, regardless of whether the entity bills Medicare for the service.[4]

If there is an ownership or compensation relationship between a physician and an entity that provides DHS, then the relationship must fit within one of the exceptions under Stark law if the treatment of Medicare patients is involved. Some Stark law exceptions include:

- Physician services[5];

- In-office ancillary services[6];

- Rental of office space[7];

- Rental of equipment[8]; and

- Personal service arrangements.[9]

The Stark law can impact physician compensation arrangements, such as productivity bonuses and profit sharing, when a physician group intends to provide DHS within its practice and to base physician compensation on DHS revenue. If a group practice wishes to distribute DHS revenue to its physicians, the group must follow several steps.

First, the group must structure the delivery of the DHS to fit within a Stark law exception. For example, a group practice that wishes to provide DHS in-house to Medicare patients usually looks to structure the delivery of the DHS to comply with the in-office ancillary services (IOAS) exception.

One of the requirements of the IOAS exception is that the physician group must satisfy the Stark law definition of "group practice." In general, a Stark law group practice must meet the following requirements:

- It must be a "single legal entity;"

- It must have at least two physicians who are members of the group;

- Each physician member must furnish substantially the full range of patient care services that the physician routinely provides through the joint use of shared office space, facilities, equipment, and personnel;

- Substantially all (defined as at least 75 percent in the aggregate) of the services of the group's member physicians must be furnished through the group and billed for under the group's billing number;

- The group practice must determine methods of distribution of overhead expenses, and income derived from the group must be distributed before receiving payment for the services giving rise to the overhead expense or producing the income;

- No physician members of the group may receive, directly or indirectly, compensation based on the volume or value of his or her referrals for DHS, except as provided with regard to productivity bonuses and profit shares, discussed below;

- Members of the group must personally conduct no less than 75 percent of the physician–patient encounters of the group; and

- Physicians in the group may be paid a share of overall profits of the group and/ or a productivity bonus, provided that the group meets certain conditions, as discussed more fully in the next section.

Group practices must meet other criteria to fit within the IOAS exception, such as who performs the DHS, who supervises the DHS, where the DHS are provided, and who bills for the DHS. Each of these criteria is detailed in 42 CFR § 411.355(b); group practices should consult legal counsel to ensure they meet the IOAS exception criteria. Assuming the IOAS criteria are met, the group practice can explore distributing DHS revenue from the practice using the Stark law special rules for productivity bonuses and profit sharing.

Stark Law Special Rules for Productivity Bonuses and Profit Sharing

Productivity Bonuses

A physician in a group practice that performs or bills for DHS may earn productivity bonuses for services he or she has personally performed or for services "incident to" such personally performed services, or both. However, the bonus must not be determined in any manner that is *directly* related to the volume or value of referrals of DHS by the physician.[10] A productivity bonus will be deemed not to relate directly to the volume or value of DHS referrals if one of the following conditions is met:

1. The bonus is based on the physician's total patient encounters or relative value units (RVUs);

2. The bonus is based on the allocation of the physician's compensation attributable to the services that are not DHS payable by a federal healthcare program or private payer; or

3. Revenues derived from DHS are less than 5 percent of the group practice's total revenues, and the allocated portion of those revenues to each physician in the group practice constitutes 5 percent or less of his or her total compensation from the group practice.[11]

These three methods are safe harbors, not requirements, and therefore a group practice is not required to meet them. The advantage of using a safe harbor is that it provides assurance that the productivity bonus is not directly related to referrals. However, a group practice may choose another method for distributing a productivity bonus as long as the method is "reasonable, objectively verifiable, and indirectly related to referrals of DHS."[12]

Even though a physician cannot tie his or her productivity bonus directly to the volume or value of DHS referrals by the physician to other providers, Stark law permits a productivity bonus to relate directly to DHS referrals for services "incident to" the physician's personally performed services.

"Incident to" services and supplies must meet the following conditions:

- They are furnished in a noninstitutional setting to noninstitutional patients (such as service outside a hospital to an outpatient);

- They are integral, though incidental, parts of the service of a physician (or other practitioner) in the course of diagnosis or treatment of an injury or illness;

- They are commonly furnished without charge or included in the bill of a physician (or other practitioner);

- They must be of a type that is commonly furnished in a physician's office;

- They must be furnished under the direct supervision of a physician (i.e., the physician must be present in the office suite but not necessarily in the same room where the services are being provided); and

- They must be furnished by the physician or a person acting under the supervision of a physician (or other practitioner).[13]

If all of the requirements set forth above are satisfied, a group practice can distribute DHS revenue through a productivity bonus based on a formula that provides physicians credit for each physician's personal productivity as well as DHS referrals for services incident to that physician's personally performed services.

Profit Sharing

Group practices are generally not permitted to distribute profits derived from DHS referrals. However, the Stark law permits "overall profit" distribution to a physician if the distribution is not determined in any manner that is directly related to the volume or value of referrals of DHS by the physician. *Overall profits* can mean either: (1) the group's entire profits derived from DHS payable by Medicare or Medicaid; or (2) the profits derived from DHS payable by Medicare or Medicaid of any component of the group practice that consists of at least five physicians.[14]

The second definition permits a group practice to create one or more subsets of the group, so long as each subset contains at least five physicians. After the DHS profits are divided among the subsets, the physicians within the subsets can be paid a share of the profits accruing to the subsets, consistent with the Stark law regulations as described herein. In other words, the group could create subsets based on specialty or location, but groups of five or more physicians should not be established based on the amount of referrals made by them to the group. The subsets could make decisions about compensating physicians within the subset, but these decisions would need to be reviewed and approved by the group's governing body.[15]

As with productivity bonuses, the Stark law creates three safe harbors for group practices to feel assured that the DHS profit shares are not "directly related" to the volume or value of referrals of DHS by the physician. Groups can adopt any of the following three safe harbors:

1. The group's profits are divided per capita (e.g., per member of the group or per physician in the group);

2. The revenues derived from DHS are distributed based on the same distribution that the group uses to distribute revenues from services that are not DHS payable by any federal healthcare program or private payer; or

3. Revenues derived from DHS constitute less than 5 percent of the group practice's total revenues, and the allocated portion of those revenues to each physician in the group practice constitutes 5 percent or less of his or her total compensation from the group.

If the group distributes profits under one of these three methods, then the group can have more confidence that their profit-sharing methodology will not come under scrutiny. However, the group may adopt other methods as long as the method of profit distribution is reasonable and verifiable and does not directly relate to the volume or value of the physician's referrals of DHS.[16]

It is important to create supporting documentation verifying the method used to calculate the profit share or productivity bonus and the resulting amount of compensation. It is possible that regulators may ask for such documentation during an investigation or audit.[17]

Anti-Kickback Statute

Similar to the Stark law, the Federal Anti-Kickback Statute (AKS) aims to deter any inclination to generate federal health program revenue through improper referrals. Three key differences between the AKS and Stark law are:

1. The Stark law is a "strict liability" law, whereas the AKS factors in a person's intent in violating the law;

2. Stark law requires the involvement of a physician in the transaction, whereas the AKS applies to "anyone;" and

3. Stark law is restricted to referrals involving Medicare, whereas the AKS applies to transactions involving any federal healthcare program.

The AKS is found at section 1128B of the Social Security Act. The implementing regulations are found at 42 CFR § 1001.951 et seq. "The anti-kickback statute makes it a criminal offense to knowingly and willfully offer, pay, solicit, or receive any remuneration to induce or reward referrals of items or services reimbursable by federal health care programs."[18] "Remuneration" includes the transfer of anything of value, in case or in kind, directly or indirectly, covertly or overtly.[19]

"The statute has been interpreted to cover any arrangement where **one purpose** of the remuneration was to obtain money for the referral of services or to induce further referrals"[20] [emphasis added]. Some safe harbor regulations define practices that are not subject to the AKS because such practices would be unlikely to result in fraud and abuse.[21] If one meets each of the conditions in the safe harbors, the entity is assured of not being prosecuted or sanctioned. Unlike Stark law, however, where failure to meet an exception automatically means one is in violation of Stark law, failure to meet an AKS safe harbor does not mean the AKS is violated.[22] Parties may reduce risk of violation by structuring arrangements to reduce improper referrals.

One important safe harbor for purposes of structuring physician compensation arrangements is the Employment Safe Harbor. Amounts paid by an employer to an employee for the furnishing of any item or service for which payment may be made in whole or in part under a federal healthcare program do not constitute prohibited "remuneration."[23,24] Generally, an employee is subject to the direction and control of the employer, receives his or her work income from the employer, and has agreed to participate in such a relationship with the employer.

The safe harbor does not limit how an employer may pay an employee. As a result, any form of compensation to employees should be acceptable. To the extent that a group practice has physician compensation arrangements to nonemployees, the group practice should structure the compensation to meet another safe harbor, if possible, such as the Personal Services and Management Contracts Safe Harbor, found at 42 CFR § 1001.952(d). Unlike the Employment Safe Harbor, the Personal Services and Management Contracts Safe Harbor contains more restrictions on the compensation paid to an "agent," such as a contractor. For example, the Personal Services and Management Contracts Safe Harbor requires that the total compensation paid to a contractor over the term of the agreement to be set in advance, consistent with fair market value in arm's-length transactions and to not be determined in a manner that takes into account the volume or value of any referrals or business otherwise generated between the parties for which payment may be made by a federal healthcare program.[25] This safe harbor is often used by hospitals, or device or pharmaceutical companies, when contracting with physicians to provide medical director or consulting services, for example. A contractor has greater independence than an employee, may have more than one clinic or hospital for whom he or she provides services, and takes on the associated risks or costs of that status, like a locum tenens.

Accountable Care Organizations

Under the Patient Protection and Affordable Care Act's (PPACA's) triple aim to achieve better health, better care, and lower costs, accountable care organizations (ACOs) take center stage. ACOs have many forms, including hospital/physician joint ventures, physician-owned ACOs, health plan/provider ACOs, and retail pharmacy-owned ACOs, for example. ACOs can also be part of the Medicare Shared Savings Program (MSSP), established by the PPACA, or they can be created by private payers. According to some 2013 reports, between 37 million and 43 million patients have physicians in ACO arrangements with at least one payer and that, including MSSP ACOs, there are 428 ACOs in 49 states and the District of Columbia. Physician groups are leading the way in forming ACOs.

Regardless of the form of ACO, the premise behind the arrangement is to promote accountability for a patient population, coordinate patient care between various providers, and incentivize higher value care. Offering financial incentives to provide higher value care is at odds with the current pay-for-volume system. Many physician compensation arrangements, including bonuses and profit sharing, are based on the pay-for-volume system. Thus, adoption of ACO models will likely require unwinding of current physician compensation agreements and replacing those agreements with methods of compensation that use performance metrics based on quality and patient satisfaction, rather than dollars in the door.

MSSP Waivers

For ACOs within the MSSP, the financial incentives to provide higher value care will likely stem from "shared savings," which are monies paid to an ACO that meets quality performance standards and demonstrates that it has achieved savings against a benchmark established by the Centers for Medicare & Medicaid Services (CMS).[26]

MSSP participants benefit from regulatory waivers issued by CMS and the Office of Inspector General (OIG) of the Department of Health and Human Services. These waivers relieve MSSP ACOs from complying with Stark law, the federal AKS, and the gainsharing Civil Monetary Penalties law.[27] Notably, however, a waiver of a specific fraud and abuse law is not needed for an arrangement to the extent that the arrangement: (1) does not implicate the specific fraud and abuse law; or (2) implicates the law, but either fits within an existing exception or safe harbor, as applicable, or does not otherwise violate the law.[28] Thus, physician compensation arrangements within an ACO that are structured to comply with the Stark law or AKS do not need a waiver from those laws, but it is likely that those arrangements may need to change to align with the ACO mission of delivering value-based care.

Because of the value-based mission of an ACO arrangement, an important waiver for purposes of physician compensation in an MSSP ACO is the Shared Savings Distribution Waiver. The intent of this waiver is to protect arrangements created by the distribution of shared savings *within* an ACO that qualifies for the waiver, as well as arrangements created by the use of shared savings to pay parties *outside*, such as an ACO if those payments are reasonably related to the purposes of the MSSP.[29] The waiver permits shared savings to be distributed or used within the ACO in any form or manner, including "downstream" distributions or uses of shared savings funds between or among the ACO, its ACO participants, and its ACO providers/suppliers.[30]

To qualify for the waiver, the MSSP ACO must meet the following conditions:

- The ACO has entered into a participation agreement with CMS to participate in the MSSP and remains in good standing under the agreement.

- The shared savings are earned by the ACO through the MSSP.

- The shared savings are earned by the ACO during the term of its participation agreement, even if the actual distribution or use of the shared savings occurs after the expiration of that agreement.

- The shared savings are either:

  - Distributed to or among the ACO's participants, its providers/suppliers, or individuals and entities that were its ACO participants or its ACO providers/suppliers during the year in which the shared savings were earned by the ACO; or

- Used for activities that are reasonably related to the purposes of the MSSP.

- Payments of shared savings distributions made directly or indirectly from a hospital to a physician are not made knowingly to induce the physician to reduce or limit medically necessary items or services to patients under the direct care of the physician.

Thus, as long as all the above conditions are met, the MSSP ACO may distribute the shared savings to participants, like physicians, as a reward for meeting the ACO's goals, for example. In addition, the waivers issued by CMS for MSSP ACOs eliminate the burden of fair market value related to the distribution of shared savings. For example, most healthcare regulations require payments to be at fair market value, which often requires a provider to perform market research by themselves or through a consultant to determine what payment is "fair" in today's marketplace for the product or service at issue. Eliminating the burden of fair market value eliminates the need to perform such an analysis. Although this adds some flexibility in structuring physician compensation models under the MSSP, ACO participants should also be aware of IRS guidance for tax-exempt organizations participating in the MSSP, as discussed in the following section.

Special Issues for Tax-Exempt Organizations in ACOs

The IRS confirms that tax-exempt organizations can participate in the MSSP as long as their participation does not result in their net earnings going to the benefit of private shareholders or individuals, and their participation in the ACO does not result in an organization being operated for the benefit of private parties participating in the ACO.[31] For example, the IRS would likely disapprove of a tax-exempt organization that gave a board of directors excessive compensation from revenues that are meant to benefit the community. The IRS has indicated that it will not consider a tax-exempt organization's participation in the MSSP to result in impermissible private benefit when distributing shared savings where the ACO has been structured in accordance with these five factors:

1. The terms of the tax-exempt organization's participation in the MSSP (including its share of shared savings or losses and expenses) are set forth in advance in a written agreement negotiated without any conflicts of interest.

2. CMS has accepted the ACO into, and has not terminated the ACO from, the MSSP.

3. The tax-exempt organization's share of economic benefits derived from the ACO (including its share of shared savings payments) is proportional to the benefits or contributions the tax-exempt organization provides to the ACO. In other words, the tax-exempt organization that participates in an ACO should receive no more financial benefit than what it contributed to the ACO (i.e.,

there should be no excessive gains experienced by the tax-exempt organization compared to the amount it invested).

4. The tax-exempt organization's share of the ACO's losses (including its share of shared losses) does not exceed the share of ACO economic benefits to which the tax-exempt organization is entitled.

5. All contracts and transactions involved with the ACO are at *fair market value* [emphasis added].[32]

Not all five factors are required to prevent impermissible private benefit.[33]

These five factors by the IRS serve as the best guidelines for physician compensation under an ACO that is itself a tax-exempt organization or is comprised of tax-exempt participants, and these should be considered by ACO developers relative to tax-exempt organizations in determining the distribution of shared savings.

ACO Shared Savings Distribution Considerations

The MSSP regulations provide little guidance as to how to distribute shared savings to ACO participants. However, one requirement of the MSSP rules is that the ACO declares, as part of the MSSP application, how it plans to use shared savings payments, including the criteria it plans to use for distributing shared savings among the ACO participants and providers.[34] Thus, decisions regarding physician compensation may be subject to input from sources outside the employment relationship.

To the extent an MSSP ACO receives shared savings, those dollars may go through several rounds of distribution before being part of a physician's compensation package. CMS estimates that starting an MSSP ACO will cost approximately $580,000, and $1.27 million in ongoing annual costs.[35] These costs will likely include investments in health information technology and the hiring/training of care coordination personnel. To the extent that there are outstanding expenses relating to these investments, or needs to improve the ACO's ability to capture and analyze data, enhance reporting, improve facilities, or hire additional care coordinators and support staff for the ACO to enhance patient care and transition, the ACO may decide to use a portion of the shared savings for those purposes.

For the portion of shared savings that the ACO will distribute to participating providers and that will be part of the physician's compensation, it is imperative that the ACO collaborate and communicate with those physicians to ensure success with the distribution process. In creating a distribution methodology, the ACO should recognize the relative contributions of provider classes and individual providers toward ACO shared savings through efficiencies, quality, and performance. Provider classes may be carved out as follows: hospitals, primary care physicians (PCPs), and specialists. The ACO may apportion shared savings to these provider classes in percentages allocated broadly to each provider class, such as 30 percent to hospitals, 40 percent to PCPs, and 30 percent to specialists.

Regardless of the percentage allocation, the apportionment of shared savings distributed to the provider class should consider factors such as the ability of the provider class to:

- Have an impact on coordinating patient care;

- Effectively control costs;

- Successfully manage the care of the patient population and achieve desired clinical outcomes; and

- Effectively coordinate patient transitions and communicate critical patient information across all provider classes.

These factors in apportionment will likely place a higher value on PCPs than specialists because the PCP is in a better position to manage costs and coordinate care. As a result, physician compensation considerations in an ACO is likely to be vastly different than in a traditional fee-for-service model, where specialist compensation may reflect the specialist's ability to generate higher revenue for the medical group.

Once an ACO determines a provider class allocation percentage, the ACO must evaluate each individual provider's role in achieving the shared savings and his or her financial and qualitative contributions toward the ACO's goals. To effectively evaluate each individual provider, the ACO should establish a "scorecard" for each provider. The scorecard may incorporate the 33 quality measures identified by the MSSP, as well as other measures that the ACO deems appropriate.[36] However, assigning too many measures to a provider's scorecard may lead to unnecessary administrative complexity and increased opportunities for failure. Regardless of which measures the ACO includes in its scorecard, the measures should focus on quality and cost savings rather than volume.

End Notes

1. 42 CFR 411.350(a).
2. See 42 CFR § 411.354(a) (defining *financial relationship*) and 42 CFR § 351 (defining *DHS* and *entity*).
3. 42 CFR § 411.351.
4. Ibid.
5. 42 CFR § 411.355(a).
6. 42 CFR § 411.355(b).
7. 42 CFR § 411.357(a).
8. 42 CFR § 411.357(b).

9. 42 CFR § 411.357(d).

10. 42 CFR § 411.352(i)(3).

11. Ibid.

12. 42 CFR § 411.352(3); 66 *Fed. Reg.* at 909–910.

13. 42 CFR § 410.26(b).

14. 42 CFR § 411.352(2).

15. 42 CFR § 411.352(f).

16. 42 CFR § 411.352(2).

17. See 42 CFR § 411.352(4).

18. Office of Inspector General (OIG) Advisory Opinion 03-13, at 3 (June 23, 2003).

19. Ibid. at 4.

20. Ibid.

21. See 42 CFR § 1001.952.

22. OIG Advisory Opinion 97-5, at 7 (Oct. 6, 1997).

23. The employment safe harbor applies the same definition of *employee* as the Internal Revenue Code (IRC). The IRC defines *employee* as including any officer of a corporation or individuals who, under the usual common law rules applicable in determining the employer–employee relationship, has the status of employee (26 USC § 3121(d)). According to the Internal Revenue Service, common law employees are those whom you can control as to what they do and how they do it. See e.g., http://www.irs.gov/Businesses/Small-Businesses-&-Self-Employed/Employee-(Common-Law-Employee).

24. 42 CFR § 1001.952(i).

25. 42 CFR § 1001.952(d)(5).

26. See IRS Fact Sheet, Tax-Exempt Organizations Participating in the Medicare Shared Savings Program through Accountable Care Organizations, FS-2011-11 (Oct. 20, 2011).

27. See 76 *Fed. Reg.* 67992, 67993 (Nov. 2, 2011).

28. Ibid. at 67994.

29. Ibid. at 68005.

30. Ibid.

31. See note 26 above.

32. Ibid.

33. Ibid.

34. 42 CFR § 425.204(d).

35. 76 *Fed. Reg.* 67969 (Nov. 2, 2011).

36. See, for example, http://www.cms.gov/Medicare/Medicare-Fee-for-Service-Payment/sharedsavingsprogram/Quality_Measures_Standards.html.

CHAPTER 7

Plan Design, Approval, and Implementation

Step 5 Continued: Size Up the Alternatives

After reviewing alternative methodologies and options for including value-based incentives and internal practice issues, the compensation committee is ready to draft a new compensation plan. The committee starts by selecting the basic foundation that best aligns with the organizational culture and mission, and the goals of the plan. The committee will modify the basic foundation to suit practice-specific factors and then incorporates appropriate incentives to encourage and reward desired behavior, whether productivity or value based. Issues such as part-time schedules, ancillary services revenue, leadership, and citizenship activities should also be considered and included.

If value-based incentives are introduced for the first time, it is best to start with a small percentage of total compensation and increase the percentage after physicians become accustomed to the concept. As the health system migrates to value- and risk-based reimbursement, then compensation methods can follow.

During this development process, the administrator or financial manager should run some initial numbers to determine how the concept will impact the group's financial viability or if individual compensation will be drastically affected. The plan should be adjusted to keep total compensation within healthy financial numbers. Typically, a good test is to use recent actual compensation and productivity numbers, a year's worth or at least six months annualized, and run them through the proposed formula. Look for issues related to internal and external benchmarks, market compensation, equity, and large positive or negative individual changes that might create problems. Remember, it is probable the entire compensation pie may not change, but the size of the individual slices of the pie will. The committee can use this period to generate ideas on how to mitigate significant impacts on physician compensation.

The committee may choose to draft more than one compensation plan to enable the committee or practice leadership to evaluate options. The committee won't want to spend time on too many options, but it can be helpful if there are issues in selecting a foundation or developing the details. Different plan options can be tested and evaluated for compliance with the group's financial goals and their impact on physician compensation.

Depending on organizational structure and culture, the committee will decide whether or not more than one option for the compensation plan will be presented. Practices that are part of health systems or academic medical centers may need to have plans approved by organizational leadership prior to releasing the concept to group physicians. Practice culture may require physician involvement in selecting from more than one option, or the committee may have the knowledge and trust to narrow the options down to one suggested design.

Best Practices in Plan Design

As the committee drafts the compensation plan(s), it should review the critical success factors to ensure they are covered. The following questions should be reviewed and answered to ensure that the plan includes organizational alignment, meets goals and objectives, and incorporates the necessary factors that should be considered:

- Is the plan in alignment with the practice's culture, mission, and vision?
- Does it align with objectives developed for the compensation plan?
- Does the plan support financial success for the organization?
- Is there sufficient financial support to reward the desired incentives?
- Does the plan encourage and reward the desired behavior: productivity, quality, outcomes, and patient satisfaction?
- Will practice leadership and citizenship activities be encouraged and adequately compensated, if appropriate?
- Have other internal issues been addressed, including part-time schedules, call coverage, support for new physicians, and so forth?
- Does the plan create accountability or at least awareness of costs and their impact on compensation?
- Will physicians have the opportunity to earn competitive compensation based on the market?
- Are the plan's goals attainable and realistic?
- Do they represent the desired mix of individual, department, and organizational goals and incentives?

- Are the goals and metrics clearly defined and understandable?

- Are goals and measures within physicians' control?

- Does the plan provide the opportunity to earn competitive compensation based on the marketplace?

- Is the plan equitable? Will the desired goals and provider efforts be valued and rewarded in a fair manner?

- Is the plan simple enough to be understood but complex enough to address all the necessary issues and challenges?

- Is the plan aligned with the reimbursement systems of the major payers? Can it be adjusted if reimbursement systems are modified?

- Are the sources of benchmarking data and value-based measures trusted?

- Will physicians be able to game the system to increase their compensation? Will it encourage upcoding, unbundling, creative coding, unnecessary procedures, or repeat visits? What are the checks and balances to minimize gaming?

- Is there a reliance on objective measures while minimizing subjective measures?

- Will external data be received in a timely manner to determine incentives or final compensation?

- Does the plan comply with all applicable regulations and laws?

- Can changes resulting from plan implementation be tracked to ensure that objectives are met?

- Is the plan reasonable to administer or will additional staff be required to run a very complex formula?

Testing Draft Compensation Plans

Before finalizing the compensation plan, it should be tested to identify any potential issues and ensure that it meets the financial expectations as indicated earlier in this chapter. Modeling will identify some, but not all, of the potential outcomes of the plan's implementation. Actual practice data should be entered in the formula to evaluate results on the practice's financial performance, and total and individual physician compensation.

The model should be tested with different variables to ensure that it has the resilience and flexibility needed. One variable to test is changes in physician behavior in response to the incentives. Plan developers may be assuming that physicians will respond in a specific manner, but alternative responses should be considered and included in the testing. Physicians may respond by changing the types of procedures offered, reducing number of visits to concentrate on the quality factors, upcoding, or other changes. Additional variables to test include:

- Changes in reimbursement rates;
- Increases in new reimbursement incentives;
- Loss of a major payer or employer;
- Declines in visits or procedures; and
- Changes within the practice, including hiring new physicians, adjustments in schedules, or loss of any physicians or specialties.

The modeling also tests the group's information systems for the capability to accurately track and report data needed to support the compensation plan. Run the tests with several months' or years' worth of past data to ensure that the plan holds up as envisioned. Use the information systems or other tools to develop and test reports for sharing applicable data with the group's leadership and physicians.

If not already in use, physician performance reports or scorecards should be developed. These tools provide physicians with information to show how their compensation is determined and the measures that are used. The reports should show the various factors involved in compensation determination, including productivity measures and the three to six value-based measures used in incentive or total compensation calculation. The reports should be short, one to two pages, and easily understood. There may be two types of physician reports: one for the specific measures that are used in physician compensation and another comparing the physician's status on all quality, satisfaction, and outcomes metrics that are tracked by the group practice. These physician reports or scorecards can present only internal data or include external data. They are more effective if physicians are able to view their status compared with a large group of their peers. Reporting internal data for and to all the physicians tends to encourage the low performers to do better during the next reporting period. Exhibit 2.11 is an example of a ranking report using financial and wRVU data. Exhibit 10.1 (later in chapter 10) is an example utilizing practice-selected quality factors.

The testing period is also the time to identify any potential objections or concerns from physicians and questions or suggestions that could arise. The committee must be prepared to address as many questions or concerns that might arise and to explain the potential impact of some of the suggestions. The committee should remain open to considering new suggestions or modifying the plan if sufficient concerns are raised. However, the committee doesn't have to please everybody, and if they do, there might be something wrong with the plan.

Transition and Implementation Plan

Before presenting the final plan or plan options, the committee needs to develop a transition or implementation plan. Several options for implementation include:

1. An immediate changeover, with the old plan closing down as the next plan starts up;

2. A transition period with the new plan running parallel to the current plan for a specific time period and monthly comparisons shared with the physicians; or

3. A phased transition with portions of the new plan being introduced at different stages. For example, productivity-based incentives can be introduced initially with value-based incentives implemented later.

The option chosen will depend on the practice and the new plan. If the new plan is similar in concept to the previous plan and changes in compensation are minimal, then the immediate-changeover method will be quicker and easier to implement. It's still recommended to wait a few months after the compensation plan decision is finalized before implementing the new plan to ensure that everyone is prepared for the switch.

If the new formula is quite different than the previous one, then the transition period or phased transition options are recommended since they include a time period for physicians to become accustomed to the change. Physicians can use the opportunity to modify behavior in order to adjust and succeed under the new plan. The transition period should be long enough to provide adequate time to ease the transition but with a realistic end. Six months to one year is typically sufficient.

If there is a potential for major changes in compensation amounts, the committee and administrators should consider whether steps should be taken to minimize the impact. A transition period enables physicians to adjust their behavior prior to full implementation of the new plan. Another option is to place a cap on the amount of change in compensation that will occur, at least for the first year or two. For example, the plan can state that no one physician's compensation will decrease (or increase?) by more than 5 or 10 percent from one year to the next. For example, The Southeast Permanente Medical Group in Atlanta, Ga., offered guaranteed salaries for three years with no greater than a 10 percent decrease in compensation in any one year when it changed from salary-based compensation to a pay-for-performance (P4P) plan.[1]

Step 6: Present the Information

After the plan has been sufficiently tested, it is ready to be presented to the group. Schedule a meeting that is dedicated to the topic and will be attended by the maximum number of physicians in the group or department. Consider scheduling the meeting outside of clinical hours to ensure greater attendance. Several days before the meeting, key information can be distributed to provide physicians with an opportunity to review the background information and basic design concepts. These materials should reiterate the reasons for the needed change and present enough information to provide a preview of the general concepts and objectives without alarming the physicians. It is not recommended to provide individual physician compensation information at this point. The physicians who are losing compensation will ignore the logic of the new plan and only focus on their losses.

A physician member of the committee should take the lead as the author of the initial materials and lead presenter. Physicians in the group are more likely to accept the plan if a peer is seen as leading the effort.

Begin the presentation with the group's leadership describing the background information on how the practice compares to nationwide financial, quality, and patient satisfaction data. The opportunities or need for financial improvement should be discussed along with the agreed-upon mission and goals of the compensation committee and plan. Leadership should introduce the committee to show their support of the committee and its plan. Consultants or other outside, objective voices, such as an accountant who participated in plan development, should contribute to the presentation. A financial officer or accountant can also explain the current financial situation and impact of the plan's implementation.

Present the recommended plan, how it works, and why it is recommended. Describe why this plan was chosen over other compensation foundations and how it addresses financial and other issues in the practice. Explain the plan as simply as possible to minimize confusion. Use data reports, spreadsheets, diagrams, and so on, to help physicians visualize details of the new plan.

Clearly define and explain new factors in determining compensation, including quality measures, costs, outcomes, and patient satisfaction scores, and why these factors are being included. List the source of the data and who is responsible for tracking it. Physicians should be allowed to ask questions at this point to ensure that the measures are clearly understood as well as paths to achieve the goals. It is important to gain physician trust of the data and an understanding of the metrics and how they can be achieved. Include the difference between individual and team goals, and who the "team" is that will be striving toward achieving goals and rewards.

Demonstrate that the practice has the data collection and reporting capability to support the new model. Present the spreadsheet for entering practice data used in compensation calculation. Discuss the flexibility of the plan to adjust to changes in practice activity during the year along with changes in reimbursement incentives. At this point, share an example of the physician reports or scorecards and general information about the potential impact on compensation. Physician-specific scores and details on compensation should be presented privately and only after the objectives and concepts are presented and hopefully agreed to.

The consultant and committee will discuss the transition and implementation plan including when implementation will begin and how a transition period or phased transition will occur. Discuss how physicians will receive reports tracking their compensation. The implementation date should be a few months from the presentation date to enable physicians to prepare and to track physician compensation and practice financial performance under the new plan. Describe the support and changes in operations or infrastructure that will be implemented to assist physicians in meeting the goals before and after implementation.

Allow plenty of time for questions and answers. If a physician asks, "What if...?," the financial representative or administrator should be ready to enter the "what if" numbers in the spreadsheet to show the potential impact. When physicians offer suggested changes, explain whether those options were considered and why they were not included. However, the committee should remain open for including options that were not considered and those that a majority of physicians are in favor of that could improve the plan.

Physician Reports or Scorecards

Physician-specific numbers can be shared during the meeting by distributing letters or reports in sealed envelopes, or the committee or group leadership could announce when private meetings will be scheduled. Individual meetings are usually recommended. When the reports are shared with physicians, there should be an opportunity to discuss and ask questions to ensure that physicians understand the reports and data points, and everyone trusts the data. These reports should be accompanied with materials to clearly describe the metric and how the data was tracked and gathered. The presenter can describe the reports and the results and be ready to address any challenges to the data. The private meetings can also be used to provide specific information to physicians who will need more support to achieve expected improvements toward compensation goals. Offer suggestions on how productivity can be increased or what techniques can be used to improve value-based metrics. Consider offering additional training or education along with staff or mentor support.

The scorecards or reports should continue to be confidential, although physicians can be encouraged to share results. The competitive nature of physicians often encourages self-improvement when faced with comparative data. Physician scorecards should be offered on a regular basis, at least quarterly, and many practices encourage physicians to view their reports at any time through secure Websites. Individual information can sometimes be kept confidential by using "blinded data," assuming the number being reported on is large enough.

Step 7: Determine the Outcome

After completion of the presentation and distribution of reports to individual physicians, the committee should consider making modifications based on physician input during and after the presentation based on the quality of the suggestions and their impact on physician compensation and the group's financial viability. If modifications are included, the final plan should be distributed to physicians for additional review. Provide a specific period of time, (i.e., in one week or by the next Monday) for physicians to provide comment. The spreadsheet for compensation calculation and physician reports should be modified to incorporate the changes.

Physicians may not be excited about the plan and may be hesitant to approve it, so it may be necessary to explain that the plan may seem unfair but is equally unfair as well. Reiterate that the current financial situation and changing healthcare environment are requiring that changes be implemented, and that all physicians in the practice will be impacted with the change. A variety of counseling and change management techniques may be required to persuade physicians to see the need for the new compensation formula. The committee can explain how a review will be conducted six months or one year after implementation to evaluate the effectiveness of the plan and for physicians to provide additional input.

The vote for accepting the new compensation plan will occur following guidelines in the by-laws. If approved, the date for implementation should be set. If not approved, the practice leadership and compensation committee should decide whether modifications are needed to gain acceptance or if the process should be started over. By gaining input from physicians and conducting the process with openness and transparency, hopefully the latter should not be the case. Some practices will require a "super majority" or greater than 50 percent approval vote to pass a new compensation plan. This should be taken into consideration if it appears a small block of physicians can and will vote against the plan to protect their self-interest. It is best to address their issues in advance of the vote, if possible.

Implementation

Value-based incentive compensation can be distributed as part of a physician's regular compensation, but a greater impact may be made if incentive payments are distributed separately. This option enables physicians to see the specific amounts of compensation as a result of their performance related to quality-based activities separate from productivity- or salary-based compensation. Incentive payments should be shared biannually, although physician scorecards should be available monthly. Separate distribution of incentive payments may be the only option if they are dependent on the receipt of incentive-based reimbursement or shared savings distributions that occur after a delayed period. If this is the case, physicians will need reminders through the year on how their behavior is contributing to the group's effort to win these incentives. As a general rule, the more frequent the reporting and reward distribution, the more effective the program.

Opportunities for physicians to express their concerns during pre- and post-implementation periods should be clearly described. Physicians should know the process to file complaints about the methodology and their compensation calculation as well as whom to take their complaints to. The contact will depend on the organizational structure, but it should not be the physician's direct supervisor, if possible. The medical director(s) or governing board typically serves as the contact.

Step 8: Evaluate the Impact and Outcome

After implementation, the impact of the new compensation plan should be tracked and its outcomes evaluated. Develop charts and diagrams to track the key indicators in practice financials, operations, and value-based ratings along with physician compensation. Develop easy-to-understand visuals and explanations to help physicians understand the impact. Use a variety of messaging methods to report the status of practice changes, including monthly department or group meetings, individual meetings, e-mails, and newsletters. Celebrate the progression toward goals.

Practice revenue, expenses, and compensation distribution should be monitored monthly to ensure there are no immediate unforeseen consequences or concerns. Ensure that the data tracking and reporting systems are accurate and easy to use or whether modifications are needed. Identify any errors or glaring areas of dysfunction in the plan that need to be addressed immediately. Accuracy is critical, because if errors are made, it can take a long time to earn back a physician's trust. When errors are found over time, be careful how corrections are made. Large take-backs of overpayments will create ill will and should be limited and recovered over time. Underpayments should be addressed promptly but limited to a specific amount of time for the reconciliation period, if possible.

Periodically double-check or audit the compensation plan to ensure calculation accuracy. It is much better to identify and self-disclose problems or errors than to have the issues grow and become unmanageable.

A formal review should be conducted at six months and again at one year to consider whether modifications should be made. The compensation committee or practice leadership should address the following questions to review the plan and its impact:

- Is the physician compensation model still in alignment with the practice's goals and mission?

- Did physicians respond to the plan as predicted, or are there unforeseen consequences that require refinements?

- Have external influences, including reimbursement systems, changed since the process began?

- Are practice goals and the compensation methodology still in alignment with external factors?

- Is the plan maintaining the organization's financial goals?

- Are physicians satisfied with the plan?

Along with financial indicators, the group's coding, encounter, quality, outcomes, and patient satisfaction data should be compared with the pre-implementation data and fully evaluated to determine whether there are any unexpected consequences that need to be addressed. Results of the comparison should be shared with physicians to celebrate successes and to introduce tactics to correct concerns, if needed.

Survey physicians after six months and one year to assess their satisfaction, concerns, and ideas regarding the compensation plan. Ensure that actual implementation occurred as expected. Ask physicians for ideas on improving the data-gathering and reporting mechanisms. Consider what adjustments should be made based on physician feedback.

Status reports should be shared throughout the year, but a one-year anniversary is an opportunity to evaluate the plan's success in aligning with organizational mission and the plan's goals. Administrators should review compensation plan best practices (listed at the beginning of this chapter) and assess their plan's effectiveness in addressing those questions.

Administrators should monitor progress toward goals. When they are achieved by a majority of physicians, decide whether the targets should be raised or if the measure should be removed from the compensation calculation and replaced by another. Some measures will continue to be a major factor in practice success and therefore continued as part of compensation, even if the amount of incentive payment or compensation dependent on a measure is reduced. However, the priority of other measures may be changed depending on reimbursement incentives or practice goals. Value-based measures should continue to be monitored via physician report cards even if they are no longer a factor in compensation.

Data should be evaluated to identify whether physicians are gaming the system. Coding, relative-value-unit numbers, types of procedures, and patient risk adjustment should be compared with pre-implementation baselines and external benchmarking data. If compensation incentives include patient satisfaction or patient engagement and compliance in care plans, physicians may be tempted to discharge noncompliant or sicker patients. Monitor for increasing numbers of the discharge of patients from physician panels or discharges for suspicious reasons. Offer advice and support to physicians dealing with noncompliant patients and consider hiring a patient education

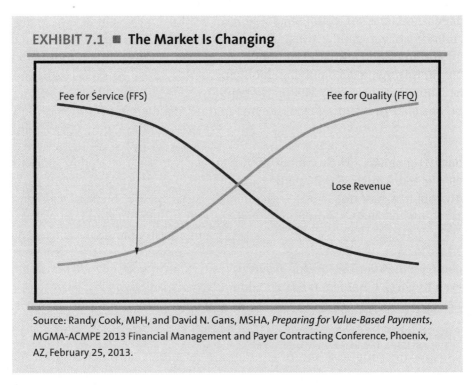

EXHIBIT 7.1 ■ The Market Is Changing

Fee for Service (FFS)

Fee for Quality (FFQ)

Lose Revenue

Source: Randy Cook, MPH, and David N. Gans, MSHA, *Preparing for Value-Based Payments*, MGMA-ACMPE 2013 Financial Management and Payer Contracting Conference, Phoenix, AZ, February 25, 2013.

specialist. Compensation methodology can be adjusted to ensure adequate incentive and reward for managing an at-risk population to counter these temptations.

After initial success within value-based reimbursement, practices need to prepare for the transition when a greater percentage of compensation is value based and the fee-for-service (FFS) revenue is declining, making it difficult to maintain total revenue (see Exhibit 7.1). David N. Gans, MGMA senior fellow, Industry Affairs, warns that the midpoint in the transition is the most difficult time for practices to succeed.[2] He bases his concern on the similar issue that practices dealt with as the marketplace shifted from FFS to capitation. In order to maintain the FFS income, Todd Evenson, director, MGMA-ACMPE Data Solutions, recommends that practices maintain incentive compensation slightly behind the shift to value-based reimbursement.[3] The compensation methodology must be flexible enough to allow an increase in value-based compensation as the FFS productivity-based share decreases.

Start Over

After struggling through the lengthy process of plan development and implementation, no one wants to hear that it's time to start over. However, the plan and its outcomes must be constantly monitored to determine when it is time to rewrite or develop a new compensation plan.

With the volatility of healthcare and reimbursement in today's environment, no one can sit back and rest. Along with preparing for changes in the amount of reimbursement dependent on new systems, groups must be willing to adjust to totally new reimbursement methods. The current systems are too new for payers to identify the best practices and most effective methods and to know whether they are having the expected impact. Current methods are being modified and new pilot programs and ideas introduced. The systems are also too new for medical groups to understand the most effective compensation and incentive formulas to respond to the new reimbursement methods.

Be prepared to adjust as the industry adjusts. Keep abreast of changes and ideas by attending conferences and webinars, monitoring the MGMA and other Websites, reviewing literature, and learning from peers and consultants. Keep your eyes and ears open for new ideas on structuring physician compensation and incentive systems, and prepare to share and implement them. Return to chapter 1 for reminders on when the plan should be reviewed and rewritten or the process started again.

End Notes

1. Willie F. Rainey Jr., MD, and Chrissy Van Erkelens, RN, "Genuine Quality and Service Incentives in a Physician P4P Program," *Group Practice Journal*, 59, no.8 (2010): 21, 24, 26–27.
2. David N. Gans, "Preparing for Value-Based Payment" (presentation at MGMA 2013 Financial Management and Payer Contracting Conference, Phoenix, AZ, February 25, 2013).
3. Todd B. Evenson, "New Trends in Physician Compensation Planning," MGMA webinar, April 18, 2013.

CHAPTER 8

Integrated Physicians and Integrated Compensation: Hospital and Health System Employed Physicians

Nick A. Fabrizio, PhD, FACMPE, FACHE, and Mary Mourar, MLS

Goals for Integration

Physicians and hospitals are uniting at an increasing rate. Physician recruitment firm Merritt Hawkins' search assignments show the trend (Exhibit 8.1) with 64% of the assignments in 2012 for hospitals or health systems.[1]

There are many reasons behind the driving integration, and physicians and hospitals may have different reasons or perspectives for affiliating. Hospitals frequently pursue integration with physicians for the following reasons:

- Achieve clinical integration to improve patient care and achieve cost savings to match changing reimbursement incentives;

- Participate in payer's alternative care or accountable care organization (ACO) programs;

- Increase their position in the marketplace to compete more effectively;

- Decrease competition with independent practices and physicians;

- Offer new services or needed subspecialty services;

- Improve call coverage;

- Increase market share;

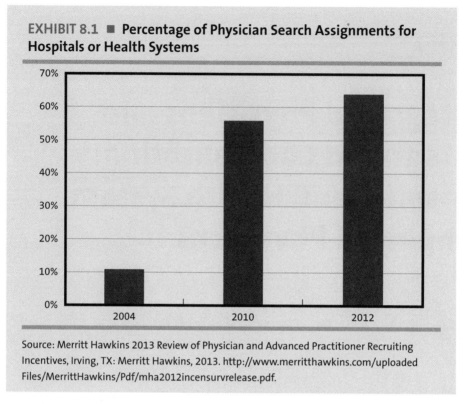

EXHIBIT 8.1 ■ Percentage of Physician Search Assignments for Hospitals or Health Systems

Source: Merritt Hawkins 2013 Review of Physician and Advanced Practitioner Recruiting Incentives, Irving, TX: Merritt Hawkins, 2013. http://www.merritthawkins.com/uploaded Files/MerrittHawkins/Pdf/mha2012incensurvrelease.pdf.

- Prevent competitors from employing physicians;
- Secure referral base; and/or
- Increase revenue from physicians' services and ancillary services.[2]

Physicians have their own reasons to seek integration or employment with health systems including:

- Stable, more secure compensation;
- Improved quality of life;
- Support in administrative and regulatory complexity;
- Investment in technology and information systems;
- Decrease in the administrative burdens of practice management;
- Receiving Medicare or private payer's shared savings or other incentive payments; and
- Accepting better compensation and benefit packages than a private practice can offer.

Hospitals and physicians use a variety of affiliation options, from call coverage and medical director agreements to joint ventures and fully integrated employment models

EXHIBIT 8.2 ■ Physician–Hospital Affiliation and Integration Options

Level of Affiliation	Option
Lowest	Call coverage
	Medical directorship
	Joint ventures
	Management service organizations
	Accountable care organizations
Highest	Employment or practice subsidiary models

(Exhibit 8.2). The many options provide physicians and systems with an opportunity to select the most appropriate model depending on their goals for affiliation and level of desired autonomy. Notice, however, that the hospital's and physician's reasons for integration are not aligned. This can make for difficult negotiation of performance and compensation expectations between physicians and health systems, as will be discussed in this chapter.

Public and private payers see the benefits of clinical integration through improved care coordination. Transfer of a patient's care from one provider or facility to another is where frequent errors are made or where providers are unable to track patients' success in following discharge planning. Medicare and private payers have implemented several reimbursement systems to encourage clinical integration and care coordination, including ACOs and bundled payments. These programs have contributed to some recent integration efforts, with participants seeking to enroll in the programs and receive shared savings or other incentive payments.

Clinical integration is achieved via "a network of interdependent healthcare facilities and providers that collaboratively develop and sustain clinical initiatives."[3] Integration involves sharing data across multiple levels of care; investing in integrated technology information systems, standardized medical best practices and processes, and increased care coordination; and aligning incentives between physicians and health systems.

Systems with the goal of increasing organizational revenue through physician-generated revenue should recognize several issues that may reduce physician revenue compared to their previous private-practice setting, including differences in:

- Physician work effort;
- System billing practices; and
- Patient population.

One difference will be physicians' work effort. Physicians may be looking to limit their clinical and administrative responsibilities in exchange for a guaranteed income.

This can be somewhat countered by basing compensation on productivity levels or incentives.

Collections per relative-value-unit (RVU) ratios may be lower than in physician-owned practices if the system uses provider-based billing, which allows systems to bill facility fees to cover the costs of locations where procedures are performed, concurrent with reductions in physician payment. The combined facility fee and reduced provider payment can be 20 percent more than the full resource-based relative value scale (RBRVS) fee paid to private practice physicians. However, doctors in the system-based group will reflect substantially less revenue on their financial statements.[4] Facilities fees may disappear in the future as payers and federal health programs decide to stop paying the additional amount.

The net collections amount per physician will also not be the same as for physicians in private practice because hospital-employed physicians frequently see more uninsured and underinsured patients. However, this may reflect the system's mission of serving the community and its citizens. Many hospital collection departments also don't emphasize collecting the smaller physicians' bills and may not have as high a collection percentage with those accounts.

Integration Models and Compensation Plans

The level of influence that health systems or integrated delivery systems (IDSs) have on physician compensation depends on the level of integration (Exhibit 8.2).[5] Models that have limited integration (medical directorships, call coverage agreements, etc.) usually involve compensation of hourly or daily stipends that are a small percentage in physicians' total compensation. Therefore, the health system's influence over total physician behavior is limited to the threat of discontinuing the contract if goals and objectives are not maintained. Hospitals and integrated systems may still incorporate quality measures expectations under these agreements.

Moderate Level of Integration

Models with a moderate level of integration may provide either a set stipend or the opportunity to achieve additional revenue, or both. Their influence on physician alignment and behavior may still be limited since the physicians' fee-for-service (FFS) revenue will have a greater influence on behavior.

Joint venture co-management and service line management agreements can include shared sharing agreements that provide physicians with a portion of incentive payments. If a sufficient amount of incentive or income is involved, physicians will see the potential financial benefits of aligning with integrated system goals and modify their behaviors. For example, a hospital participating in a bundled payment program for cardiac services wants to reduce unnecessary costs while maintaining quality. If a cardiologist increases costs by ordering redundant tests and selects expensive stents, the hospital can enter into a co-management agreement with the cardiologist. Through the agreement, in addition to the fee for professional services, the hospital can offer incentives for following protocols on recommended testing and choosing from a limited number of stent models.[6]

Hospitals or IDSs can develop management service organizations (MSOs) to provide business, human resources, and/or information technology services to physicians to increase alignment without purchasing or controlling practices. Physicians are connected through the MSO agreement and payment for the agreed-upon MSO services, but there is little link to compensation unless there are shared savings opportunities.

ACOs and systems participating in bundled payment programs can also use distribution of shared savings as incentives to encourage physicians to participate in quality and cost management goals. Exempla Healthcare in Denver, Colo., developed incentive programs based on cardiologists' average cost for mechanical valves, EKGs, and stents as part of its shared savings distribution under Medicare's Acute Care Episode demonstration program.[7]

ProHealth Solutions ACO in Waukesha, Wis., uses a pool funded by payers' incentive programs to distribute payments to affiliated physicians based on their scores in quality, efficiency or cost measures, patient satisfaction, patient safety, and access. For some specialties, there is an additional chronic care pool that encourages physicians to successfully manage more patients with chronic diseases. David Cook, chief administrative officer, meets with participating groups to encourage them to develop compensation plans in line with ACO goals.[8] This particular ACO is described in more detail in chapter 10.

High Level of Integration

The highest level of influence over physician compensation, and therefore physician behavior, is under the highest level of integration, including employment and subsidiary options. With these models, the health system has control over a larger portion (up to 100 percent) of compensation via actual remuneration or final approval of the compensation plan design. Hospitals frequently dictate how employed physicians will be compensated. Subsidiary groups may be given more leeway in developing their compensation formulas, but health system leadership approval is usually required. The optimum arrangement for determining compensation is to have hospital administrators and physicians jointly develop the compensation plan.

For the remainder of this chapter, the discussion will focus on physician compensation planning in the integration models that involve hospital employment either through the subsidiary or direct employment models. In these structures, integrated systems have the greatest influence and amount of control on compensation methodology.

Compensation Plan Design Process in Integrated Systems

There are several differences in how hospital-employed practices operate compared with private practices. To identify how those differences impact the process of physician compensation plan design, let's look again at the Decision Pathways steps.

1. Define the Problem or Opportunity

Compensation plans are developed when new physicians join the integrated system or the system realizes the current plan needs to be adjusted or a new plan developed. Systems are constantly adjusting physician compensation plans to incorporate new incentives, increase physician alignment, or adjust to changing marketplace and reimbursement influences. Reviewing current systems and physician satisfaction will always identify new opportunities for improvement. Forty-one percent of health systems and physician organizations change their physician compensation plans every one to two years according to a HealthLeaders survey.[9] Although frequent adjustments may be needed, system leaders must monitor physicians' satisfaction to ensure the adjustments aren't creating upheaval that keeps physicians uneasy or confused as to how their compensation will be determined in the future.

Just as there is no single compensation plan that is appropriate for all private practices, there isn't a "best plan" for integrated systems. System leaders must determine their goals, mission, relationships with physicians, and marketplace specifics and then develop a compensation plan that is best suited for their organization. Large systems may include a variety of physician specialties and alignment arrangements, including individual employed physicians and subsidiary groups, which may require different compensation arrangements.

Plan Goals and Objectives

Compensation plan mission and objectives should be developed that align with the organization's mission, vision, and strategic plans. This alignment is more difficult in hospital-based practices than in private practices. As stated earlier, reasons for integration often differ, leading to diverse opinions and goals for physicians and hospitals. Both parties must discuss and negotiate while contracts or integration agreements are signed to identify shared reasons and benefits for affiliation. If agreement is reached during the initial contractual phase, it will be easier to identify mutual goals for the compensation plan. This may require many meetings to come to agreement, but both parties will benefit in the long term.

Integrated systems often have prewritten or outlines of compensation plans or criteria that are used across the system. These plans should be presented to physicians during initial negotiations. If physicians are in agreement with the system's organizational mission and goals and its aligned compensation plan, then they will be more apt to support the compensation plan during their employment. Otherwise, they should not continue with the negotiation. Systems and physicians should also identify any deal breakers at the beginning of the process. However, system leadership should recognize the need to balance system standards with the need to recruit a variety of physicians. They should remain open to negotiation and flexibility in plan design if they desire to recruit more physicians.

Hospitals should prioritize their reasons for physician employment and integration and how those reasons should be reflected in the compensation formula. Physicians should also identify their priorities and what they consider to be deal breakers – items that must appear in the formula. For example, the hospital may identify that adding a new service or revenue stream is the priority, with expectations that physicians will provide an expected amount of revenue and serve an X-number of hours on call. The compensation model should then provide incentives for the physician to produce an expected amount (production) and serve the expected call schedule (expectations). The physicians' deal breaker may be that they receive adequate compensation for the call coverage (market rate) and an opportunity to earn a fair income based on their work effort.

If participating in shared savings or other value-based incentive systems is a priority of the integrated system, then physicians should be made aware of the plans for succeeding under the reimbursement systems. Hospital payment based on reducing utilization or total patient costs will provide incentives counter to the productivity-based reimbursement incentives that physicians frequently operate under. The roles and expectations for physicians to support these plans need to be shared to obtain physician buy-in. The reasons for value-based factors in incentive compensation systems should be clearly explained, along with the expected behavior to achieve the goals. Physician acceptance will be increased if they have the opportunity to provide input or select value-based measures used in the compensation or incentive formula and if incentive payments compensate for loss in FFS revenue.

Plan Designers – Committee or Not

The structure and philosophy of the integrated system will determine who develops the compensation plan and provides final approval. Physicians in subsidiary groups may develop their own compensation plan using the process and committee structure described for private practices in chapter 2. System leadership approval is usually required, so the group or plan committee should seek input from the beginning or include a system representative in the committee. The committee should compile information on organizational goals, mission, and strategic plans and if a type of compensation foundation is preferred or required. The committee should confirm at various steps in the process to ensure that plan development continues to align with system expectations.

Hospitals and IDSs that directly employ physicians may have a standard compensation plan that is presented to physicians upon hiring. Any changes in the plan can be dictated from the system leadership or compensation committee down to the physicians. However, this behavior can quickly antagonize physicians since it decreases their sense of autonomy and control. Physicians may respond with resentment and lack of full participation.

Integrated systems that incorporate physicians throughout the leadership and encourage physician participation in compensation plan design will have increased physician satisfaction, participation, and adherence to plan goals. Several options are available for including physicians in plan design that will increase physician adherence to the plan including:

1. Provide physicians with an outline of the recommended or required compensation formula and let them develop the details, which are then approved by system leadership. For example, the system may dictate that at least X percent of compensation be based on productivity and the remainder on incentives but allow the group or physicians to decide which incentive measures will be used; or

2. Include physician representation in a system-wide compensation committee. Physician buy-in will increase more if physicians vote for their representatives on the committee rather than the system leadership selecting the representatives.

System-wide compensation committees should include a representative sample of physicians to include a mix by gender, age or years with the system, and specialty. The committee should also include financial managers and legal advisors to ensure that plan development complies with financial restrictions of the organization and compliance with government regulations.

Several keys to succeeding in compensation plan negotiation include:

- Have the right people at the table;
- Share information;
- Assign physician leaders to communicate with their physician colleagues;
- Have the correct data and information;

- Ensure buy-in;

- Be transparent; and

- Don't rush the process. The average time from initial planning to implementation of the plan is 9 to 12 months.

2. Explore Information Needs

The process for identifying information needs is similar to that for private practices. The main difference is ensuring that organizational goals, mission, and plans are considered and that questions specific to hospital-employed physicians are considered. Another key difference is federal and state regulations related to physician employment and compensation, as discussed in Chapter 6, including those dealing with fair market value of total physician compensation. The committee should identify sources for legal and financial information and include a legal counselor during committee meetings and review of the drafted plan to ensure legal and regulatory compliance.

3. Collect Data

Gathering physician input at this stage is as important as it is in private practices. The more physicians who provide input into the development process, the more acceptance they will have. Survey physicians using interviews or a survey tool, similar to Exhibit 2.7 provided in chapter 2.

The literature, peer contacts, and other research should look into compensation planning in integrated and hospital-based practices as well as in private practices. The committee shouldn't limit itself in its research since ideas implemented in private practices may easily apply to their own setting. Benchmarking compensation data is especially important for hospitals because of the fair market value requirements of federal regulations to ensure that compensation offered to physicians is competitive with market rate compensation for similar services by similar organizations. Some regulations even specify the number of surveys that should be used in compensation comparison. Include reports that survey and break out data for hospital/health-system-owned practices that include most of the surveys discussed in chapter 2. The online MGMA DataDive module enables users to cross practice ownership with other factors.

Differences in how physician- and hospital-owned practices handle expense allocation, ancillary services and their revenue, and benefits will impact the figures for physician productivity and compensation as well as practice financials. Review the definitions of each data point and table in the benchmark reports and other sources to ensure that the committee is comparing apples to apples. Consider how system ownership of ancillaries and methods of expense allocation will impact physicians' revenue and compensation.

4. Interpret the Data

This step should continue as described in chapter 2.

Reviewing MGMA Physician Compensation and Production Survey data shows that hospital-based physicians often have lower income than those in physician-owned practices, perhaps due to their willingness to trade lower compensation for a reduction in hassles or an increase in quality of life. However, hospitals may also be subsidizing physician compensation since they are higher compared with collections than non-hospital-owned practices. The system's willingness to subsidize compensation may depend on competition for physicians within their marketplace and the perceived value the physician will provide to the hospital. For example, orthopedic surgeons receive higher compensation compared with collections in hospital settings than family physicians.[10]

5. Size Up the Alternatives

The compensation foundations described in chapter 3 are all options for hospital/ IDS-employed physicians. In the 1990s, hospitals frequently offered physicians a guaranteed salary and physicians accepted because one of their reasons for employment was to receive a guaranteed salary. In response, physicians emphasized their quality of life and reduced their productivity. Hospitals frequently lost money when physician-generated revenue was lower than expected and even, occasionally, lower than the guaranteed salary. Hospitals and integrated systems may be willing to subsidize compensation for specialists that support a needed service line for the hospital or community – pediatric subspecialties, for example. A guaranteed salary, or at least a guaranteed base salary, is still appropriate for these specialties. However, systems are not willing to subsidize all affiliated physicians. Integrated systems now recognize the need to specify minimum expectations for physician performance or encourage physicians to maintain or increase their productivity.

Most systems have shifted to productivity-based compensation formulas. Any of the productivity measures can be used: charges, net revenues or collections from professional services or RVUs. Collections as a productivity measure has the disadvantage of being impacted by payers' reimbursement rates and the effectiveness of the billing and collections department. Physician work RVUs (wRVUs) have the advantage of being payer blind, important in systems that have high Medicare and indigent populations, and independent of the efficiency of the collections department. If using RVUs, the plan administrators should be aware of and make adjustments for the use of modifiers and changes in RVU schedules so compensation parallels revenue, as was discussed in chapter 3. Administrators should also watch charges and collections to ensure compliance.

Compensation can be determined using a compensation per wRVU value in any of the options (set amount, tiered, or straight line increase) described in chapter 3. It is just as important to select the correct value for determining compensation. If too high a ratio is selected, the physician is rewarded with higher compensation but less money is available for the system and compensation could even exceed the compensation pool, impacting the organization's financial status. If the ratio is too low (below the median), the physicians' incentive decreases or resentment builds. Compensation per wRVU can be based on or near survey medians. Physicians will also be expecting compensation near their previous income depending on their work effort. An analysis can be conducted with current practice data to determine what compensation per wRVU value maintains compensation at near-current levels but provides incentive to increase productivity.

There are as many options for compensation formulas as there are in private practices, as discussed in chapter 3. Some of the possible methods used in integrated systems include:

- One hundred percent based on productivity (collections, charges, or a mix) minus expenses;

- Production based on compensation per wRVU value. The value can be a set amount or rise in tiers as a physician's production level increases;

- Base salary determined by production levels relative to compensation surveys. For example, if a physician's wRVU numbers match the 80th percentile of the *MGMA Physician Compensation and Production Survey* report, then the compensation is at the 80th percentile; and

- Base salary plus incentives.

Several options are available for determining the incentive payments above the base or guaranteed salary. For every wRVU above a minimum target, the physician could receive all of the RVU value as an additional reward. Another option is for the physician to be paid a percentage of the RVU value (40 to 60 percent) with the remaining percentage going to the system. The minimum production target could be based on a percentile in physician compensation and production surveys or enough revenue to cover the base salary or salary plus expenses.[11]

As described in chapter 6, physician compensation must be in compliance with several regulations to ensure that total physician compensation is within fair market value and doesn't provide direct rewards for amount or number of referrals or ancillary services (designated health services).

Incentives

Hospitals are including incentives in physician compensation plans at an increasing rate. Quality measures were included as bonuses or incentives for 35 percent of recruited positions in 2012, compared to less than 7 percent in 2010/2011, but made up less than 10 percent of the total potential bonus. More than 90 percent of physician search positions featured bonuses or compensation based on productivity, and wRVUs were the productivity measure in more than half of the descriptions.[12]

Physicians should be asked to contribute to the identification of incentives and the measures to include in compensation incentives. Physicians are also best qualified to design the quality portion of the incentive since they know their specialty and treatment protocols. Otherwise, they may resent the hospital's effort as coercion rather than a cooperative effort. Along with productivity and financial measures, incentives can be based on following supply chain standardization or treatment protocols and care guidelines, implementing cost-efficiency measures, and emphasizing patient satisfaction, as well as physicians' scores on disease management and population health management measures.

As described in other chapters, measures used in determining compensation and incentives must be clearly defined, understood, and within the control of physicians. Examples of measures within physician control include individual productivity, coding and documentation, interaction with others, quality of care, and patient satisfaction related to physician services. Employed physicians have less control over payer mix, fee schedule, developing market share, and so on.

Physicians must trust the data used in incentive determination and its source and know the behavior that is required of them to achieve the goals. All of these factors are more difficult in large integrated systems with complex information system infrastructure. Administrators must be able to track how information is entered into the system and how it is reported to reassure physicians.

Incentives related to the achievement of organizational goals or objectives can be included to encourage alignment with the organization. For example, if clinical integration and participating in shared savings programs are system priorities, then the compensation plan should include quality and cost-effectiveness incentives. Physicians can receive bonuses or incentive payments when financial goals are achieved or the organization receives shared savings payments. For example, all physicians and staff at the Henry Ford Health System in Detroit, Mich., are eligible for a bonus if their business unit meets service and budget targets, and if financial goals for the whole system are exceeded. Physicians are also eligible for a bonus if they achieve or exceed goals in quality, patient satisfaction, and prescription patterns.[13]

Participation in committees, organizational leadership, protocol development, community events, and similar factors should be considered as well. ProHealth Solutions (Waukesha, Wis.) has an excellent example of an ACO incentive system that includes incentives for system and community citizenship (described later in chapter 10).

Integrated systems can help physicians transition into the future of value-based reimbursement with physician performance reports or compensation incentives. Factoring in quality, outcomes, satisfaction, and cost-effectiveness will raise awareness of these issues and the changing reimbursement, and will support organizational goals. As reimbursement shifts more toward value-based compensation, incentives must follow accordingly but carefully. Robert C. Bohlmann, MGMA healthcare consultant, advises systems to use a slow startup and progression with adequate physician education. "Anything that smacks of a big system forcing transitions will not bode well," he warns; "physician pushback has already been observed."[14]

Use physician performance reports or scorecards to track physician numbers compared to their peers and goals for each of the measures used in calculating compensation and determining compliance with value-based measures. Scores in comparison reports can be a main influence in physician behavior since peer competition is very effective. The scorecards also keep physicians' eyes on organizational priorities and goals.

The compensation pool must be calculated to determine the amount of money available for income distribution. The pool can be generated through a combination of total hospital and system revenue, or just the revenue generated by the physician. If physicians were recruited from private practice, they were used to receiving revenue from ancillary services. Hospitals typically own ancillary services and must decide if hospital revenue should be distributed to physicians to maintain expected levels of compensation. Physicians will also view the system as a bottomless source of revenue and need to be shown that the compensation pool is still limited by revenue minus expenses. Ensuring transparency with the organization's financial status will encourage trust between physicians and system leadership.

Expense allocation is handled in different ways depending on system structure and philosophy. Physicians' direct and indirect expenses may be allocated or indirect expenses absorbed as part of total hospital or system expenses. Including cost allocation in the compensation determination will increase physicians' accountability toward the financial sustainability of their practices relative to their revenue. Allocation of physician and practice expenses is easier in the subsidiary practice model since most expenses can be identified and tracked. Direct expenses are usually allocated even for directly employed physicians. Variable expenses, such as personnel and supplies, are often fully allocated. This can be handled with equal distribution or based on a percentage of production.[15]

Administrators may want to allocate some of the system's overhead to physicians. If this is limited to a percentage of overhead related to services provided to the physician (billing, collections, human resources, staffing, etc.) then the system may be able to explain their case in a manner that is acceptable to physicians. However, if physicians believe they have no control over the expenses or are allocated expenses beyond what directly supports their activities, they may feel resentment.

6. Present the Information

The draft compensation plan should be presented to physicians during a face-to-face meeting via either individual meetings or department or system physician meetings. A physician committee member or leader should be the main presenter to encourage physician buy-in. The presentation should follow the format described in chapter 7. Presenters should be prepared to answer questions and take suggestions.

Describe the implementation and transition plan, contacts for filing complaints, and support that will be provided, if needed, to help physicians achieve the goals.

7. Determine the Outcome

Acceptance of the proposed plan may not require a vote as described for physician-owned practices, but physician acceptance of the plan is still important to maintain physician satisfaction and retention. Therefore, the committee or system leaders should obtain physician input about the plan, determine if it includes all the identified physician goals and deal breakers, and ensure physician understanding of the measures and activity that is needed to succeed under the plan. If there are major concerns or complaints, offer clear explanations or consider whether modifications are needed.

Implementation should follow the transition plan developed by the committee or system leadership. The transition period will provide physicians with an opportunity to adjust to the plan and learn what will be needed to succeed with the performance measurements. With large organizations like integrated systems, it is often difficult to determine who is the "go to" person for physicians to provide feedback and to address their questions and concerns. Contacts should be clearly identified, along with the path for filing complaints regarding compensation calculations.

8. Evaluate the Impact and Outcome

This step should proceed as described in Chapter 7. Data gathering to track progress toward organization and physician goals should be constantly monitored. Multiple information systems may be in place between the different settings within the organization. If a minor change is made in one setting, it's difficult to foresee the consequences down the line for tracking and reporting the clinical activity, costs, quality, and other measures.

Gathering physician feedback following compensation plan implementation is very important so physicians sense that their views and concerns are respected and valued in the large organization. Because of the diverse goals and objectives of the system and its physicians, monitoring the plan's continued alignment with the committee's identified goals and objectives is imperative. Evaluate whether the plan's incentives are encouraging the desired behavior needed to achieve organizational goals and mission. Physicians may want to prioritize FFS activities to maintain their income, particularly if they're subjected to productivity-based plans. However, if the organization wants to encourage citizenship and improve its scores on value-based factors, then physician behavior should be monitored to ensure that incentives included in the compensation plan are sufficient to achieve the desired results.

It is important to maintain physicians' sense of community within the organization through the compensation plan and other means. Annual or biannual physician meetings are opportunities to celebrate progression toward goals and plans for the future. The physicians' role in achieving the goals and being part of the community should be emphasized. Physician scorecards or performance reports should be distributed at the meetings, along with the check for incentive payments.

Evaluating the outcome should include monitoring the measures analyzed during the data collected and benchmarked during Steps 3 and 4 and included in physician incentive plans. If the measures don't improve or targets aren't obtained, then incentives may need to be modified or the agreement rewritten. For example, when the Iowa Health System (renamed UnityPoint Health in 2013) aligned with an orthopedic practice under a shared management company, the agreement specified the quality, production, and financial metrics for the group to achieve. The 27-physician orthopedic group had approached the health system with an option to work together more closely after it opened a new acute care facility with emphasis on orthopedics. The two partners developed a limited liability management company with shared ownership. The Iowa Health System monitored the metrics postagreement and found that the physician incentives based on decreasing lengths of stay resulted in a 30 percent decrease in length of stay for knee and hip surgery. Other incentives resulted in increased patient satisfaction scores leading to an increase in the number of patients, including some from surrounding areas.[16]

End Notes

1. Merritt Hawkins 2013 Review of Physician and Advanced Practitioner Recruiting Incentives (Irving, Texas: Merritt Hawkins, 2013), 3. http://www.merritthawkins.com/uploadedFiles/MerrittHawkins/Pdf/mha2012incensurvrelease.pdf.

2. Justin Chamblee, CPA, "Physician Compensation: Design a Plan That Responds to Integration and Alignment" (presentation at MGMA Financial Management and Payer Contracting Conference, Phoenix, AZ, February 24–26, 2013).

3. Ibid.

4. David N. Gans, "Data Mine: Why Hospital-Owned Medical Groups Lose Money," *MGMA Connexion* (April 2012), http://mgma.com/workarea/mgma_downloadasset.aspx?id=1370391 (accessed February 21, 2013).

5. See note 2 above.

6. M. Driscoll, "Physician Acquisition: What to Avoid After the Deal Is Complete," *hfm (Healthcare Financial Management)*, 66, no.4, (2012): 90–94.

7. Debbie Welle-Powell, MPA, "Beyond Fee for Service – Moving to Episodes and Bundled Payments," MGMA webinar, June 2, 2011.

8. David Cook, chief administrative officer, ProHealth Solutions (Waukesha, Wis.), personal conversation with author, March 6, 2013.

9. Karen Minich-Pourshadi, "Physician Compensation Incentives Shifting," *HealthLeaders Media* (October 28, 2011), http://www.healthleadersmedia.com/content/MAG-272014/Physician-Compensation-Incentives-Shifting.html (accessed February 17, 2013).

10. David N. Gans, "Data Mine: What Drives Physician Salaries?" *MGMA Connexion* (October 2012).

11. Nick A. Fabrizio, PhD, FACMPE, with Robert C. Bohlmann, FACMPE, *Integrated Delivery Systems: Ensuring Successful Physician–Hospital Partnerships* (Englewood, CO: Medical Group Management Association, 2010), 98–106.

12. Merritt Hawkins 2012 Review of Physician Recruiting Incentives. Press Release (July 2, 2012), http://www.merritthawkins.com/uploadedFiles/MerrittHawkins/Pdf/mha2012incensurvrelease.pdf (accessed April 22, 2013).

13. Lola Butcher, "Financial Incentives for Employed Physicians: Do They Work?" *PEJ*, 36 no.4 (2012): 18–21.

14. Robert C. Bohlmann, FACMPE, "Is Your Integration a Marriage of Equals?" *MGMA Directions* (Spring 2012), 4–5, http://www.mgma.com/WorkArea/mgma_downloadasset.aspx?id=1370965.

15. See note 11 above, pp. 96–97.

16. Karen Minich-Pourshadi, "Return to the Employed Physician," *HealthLeaders Magazine*, 13, no.8 (2010): 29–30.

CHAPTER 9

Academic Faculty Compensation Formulas

Nick A. Fabrizio, PhD, FACMPE, FACHE, and Mary Mourar, MLS

Many of the factors that affect physician activity and compensation are the same in academic settings as they are in private practice, but many of them are unique. Academic practices must watch their budgets as do private practices. Including incentives in compensation plans will encourage physicians to modify their behavior. If the organization is struggling financially, including incentives to be more clinically active will help increase revenue. Several main differences impact activities and compensation for academic-based physicians:

- Varied sources of funding that can be volatile;

- Three missions: clinical, teaching, and research;

- Complex organizational structure;

- Competing with private practicing physicians; and

- Recruitment and retention.

Funding for academic faculties' compensation comes from state funding (where available), research grants, and clinical activity. All three sources of funds are undergoing changes. State funding is suffering in most states because of restrictions on state budgets reducing support for higher education. Federal budget cuts threaten funding for research grants and federal support of direct and indirect education funding. Clinical activity funding is impacted by the changes in Medicare and private payer reimbursement. Academic medical centers (AMCs) often serve as community safety-net facilities, requiring them to accept more uninsured or underinsured patients than private practices or private integrated systems. As a result, clinical revenue may be lower for the similar amount of work compared to private practice.

The largest issue for academic practices is their triple mission. Clinical activity is similar to private practices, but teaching and research take time away from clinical activity, reducing the amount of revenue from clinical services. Teaching and research have different funding sources and different means of tracking physicians' activity levels and performance. Organizations supporting medical education and research need to determine the value they place on teaching and research and how to fund those activities versus clinical, reimbursable activities. Academic departments may also have to find physicians who "specialize" in either teaching, research, or clinical productivity, as trying to fulfill all three missions may prove too difficult for the academic faculty.

AMCs and community hospital-based teaching facilities can have very complex organizational structures. Medical staff may be treated as regular, tenured faculty and directly employed by the academic center or organized in faculty plans under contractual or partnership arrangements with the AMC. The amount of freedom and flexibility that faculty practices have varies widely. There is often variation within one organization related to the relationship between physicians and the entity. There can be one faculty plan for all affiliated physicians or variations between departments in one facility. Differences can be due to specialty versus primary care departments, the amount of emphasis on research or teaching, or when the department was formed or negotiations took place. Academic departments may be centralized or decentralized. The dean may have different levels of control that he or she exerts within the same medical school.

Different organizational relationships result in variations in accountability, compensation, and financial arrangements. Centers have different means of allocating state and tuition funds to departments and determining how research and outside funding is handled. Depending on organizational structure or philosophy, the faculty compensation methodology may be determined by the leadership of the center and passed down through departments or plans developed by the faculty must be passed up through the organization for approval.

History of Faculty Compensation

Historically, the most common method for determining compensation was base salaries usually linked to rank and tenure rather than teaching, research effort, and achievement. Salaries may have been based on market data or could have been determined in arbitrary manners, depending on when physicians were hired or how well they handled contract negotiations. Faculty received increases in compensation as they achieved tenure, moved up through department rank, or via annual merit or cost-of-living increases.

Compensation for physicians in academic settings has traditionally been lower than in private practices. The healthcare system does not fund research and teaching as high as clinical activities. Academic centers rely on physicians' interests and passion for teaching, research, and practicing in the academic environment and their acceptance of the lower compensation. Sometimes outside research will have funding tied to it that will have a direct impact on the physicians' total compensation, supplementing what they receive through clinical and teaching activities.

Over time, academic centers and departments realized that guaranteed salaries offered no incentives to increase clinical, education, or research activity. Compensation was not linked to revenue or practice financial factors, so maintaining organizational financial viability was an issue. Declines in state funding for higher education impacted the amount of general funds available to support faculty salaries. Increasing clinical activity was seen as a means of increasing revenue for the organization and departments in order to meet decreases in state, federal, and institutional funding. Participation in education and research activities could suffer with no incentive to maintain or increase participation. Many universities sought increased funding from grants and considered how to encourage physicians to increase the number of grants.

The use of guaranteed salaries has declined in favor. Fewer faculty members are offered guaranteed salaries, or the percentage of faculty total compensation that is guaranteed is lower. Factors related to physician performance are increasingly introduced in compensation formulas, including physicians' clinical, research, and teaching activities.

The statement from chapter 1 is as true in academic and teaching facilities as it is in private practice: If you've seen one compensation plan, you've seen one compensation plan. Also, the plan that is right for your practice is the one you write. Each organization is different (hospital vs. medical school based; one faculty plan vs. department-specific contracts, specialty, and primary care) and each organization is made up of unique, individual physicians. There are so many variations that each program must develop the compensation model that suits it. It is important not to rush the process, but to proceed at a pace to ensure there is buy-in and transparency. Given the right amount of time and inclusion in the process, the right model for the practice will be developed.

Faculty Compensation Plan Development

Plan development should occur in a methodical process similar to the development process used in private practices and described in chapter 2. This process benefits from physician input and buy-in during the process and with the final plan. However, the relationship between faculty and organization will affect how the process for developing a plan occurs. The contract and relationship will determine whether the faculty is able to develop its own plan or if the administration has control. The amount of control an entity has will also be determined by the amount that it subsidizes faculty compensation.

These contracts and arrangements frequently result in academic center leadership controlling the design of compensation formulas. The process will be more successful if completed through an interactive process or with the center leadership providing guidelines and goals, and the faculty plans or departments developing the details to submit to leadership for approval.

Compensation Committee

In the interactive process, a compensation committee should be selected to develop the plan. Because of the complexity of AMCs and the variety of departments and arrangements, compensation formulas should allow for flexibility by specialty and structure of the department or faculty plan. Independent committees for each department should be allowed to develop plans for their group within the expectations or guidelines of organization-wide directives. This is especially true if quality metrics or other specialty or department-specific factors need to be included.

The committee should include a mixture of faculty and administrative personnel, including a financial or business manager. Physician members can be elected by their peers or selected by leadership to ensure a representative mix. Selection of committee members by faculty rather than the leadership will ensure greater credibility. Again, the key is to have the right people at the table, those that are seen as leaders within their group and the financial or administrative representatives that can run the numbers and impact the decisions.

The committee should review directives from the AMC and its leadership regarding compensation methodology and gather information on organizational goals, mission, and planning. As with private practices, it is imperative for the goals and objectives of the compensation plan to align with organizational goals and objectives. Physician input is important at this stage to also assist in identifying means of recognizing the three missions of the faculty plan. Transparency throughout the process will improve the acceptance of the process and developed formula. Healthcare consultants and other business experts have a role in gathering physician input, offering ideas for the compensation plan, serving as an objective voice, and guiding the negotiation.

The compensation committee should use physician input, literature research, questioning peers, and reviews of organizational mission and directives to develop the goals and objectives of the compensation plan. Sample plan goals include:

- Recruit and retain physicians;
- Recognize and reward clinical activities;

- Encourage increased participation in teaching, research, and administration;

- Increase patient satisfaction;

- Improve financial viability through increased revenue and cost management;

- Encourage collaboration, team effort, and performance;

- Inspire innovation and extra effort in the three missions; and

- Recognize and reward improved quality and outcomes.

The faculty at one large academic surgery practice chose to write and adopt guiding principles to direct their new compensation plan development. These principles are listed as follows:

1. *To value all missions – education, research, and medical service: The program design will measure and reward all three mission-critical activities.*

2. *Equity: Equitable distribution and equitable procedures are essential components of the plan.*

3. *Simplicity: Well-understood incentives work better than complicated and confusing ones. The plan should be easy to understand from the point of view of faculty members. The computation and allocation mechanisms of the plan should be easy to administer.*

4. *Comprehensiveness: The plan has to be comprehensive enough to achieve the majority of the specified objectives. Required comprehensiveness will balance the simplicity principle in terms of program design.*

5. *Flexibility: The proposed plan will provide flexibility for expected and unexpected contingencies such as maternity leave. Administrative discretions may be needed for exceptional circumstances.*

6. *Link to financial performance: Various components of the plan will need to be directly and indirectly linked to the financial performance of the department, divisions within the department, or individual faculty members to achieve the goals of the program.*[1]

Plan Alternatives and the Three Missions

Compensation Pool Determination

The committee, under guidance with the organizational leadership, must determine the amount of money available to fund faculty compensation. All of the funding sources must be considered, including state and federal government, hospital, medical school, grants, and clinical sources. How revenue is distributed to physicians can be contract dependent and must be considered. For example, does the contract require that funds go directly to one physician or department or can it be paid to the entity to distribute?

Determine how much the physicians will be expected to generate through clinical services and grant funding and how much the entity is willing to subsidize. Teaching facilities can choose to subsidize compensation through funds received from the total activities supported by the organization or by pooling all physician revenue (clinical and nonclinical) and reallocating from those with high clinical and other revenue to those who emphasize teaching and research. Specialty department revenue can contribute to primary care departments. These are some of the same issues that large multispecialty practices have. Redistributing income will generate a significant amount of anxiety and discussion that cannot be undervalued.

Because of the volatility in grant funding and clinical activity, compensation plan administrators should consider using smoothing techniques to reduce volatility in compensation. Use rolling averages with several months or years of data to determine the compensation pool and monthly compensation.

If incentive compensation will be included in the plan, the committee should decide how much compensation will be incentive based and how it will be funded. The most typical method is through withholding a percentage of total revenue. If the facility is receiving reimbursement incentives from commercial or public payers or others sources, these payments can fund an incentive pool.

Salary

After reviewing compensation options and organizational and department goals, the compensation committee may decide that maintaining the guaranteed salary is the best option for the group but the system needs tweaking. The current salaries may be too arbitrary and not in line with reality. The salary system should be reviewed comparing individual compensation and clinical and nonclinical productivity levels with compensation and productivity of other physicians within the organization and in other academic centers. Salaries should be adjusted to align with marketplace compensation and internal financial status by either of three methods or a combination of any two:

1. Utilize data from academic faculty compensation and production surveys;

2. Utilize data from private practice compensation surveys; and/or

3. Calculate the compensation pool from combined revenue minus expenses.

Salaries can be benchmarked and compared with data for similar AMCs based on faculty rank, percentage of clinical time, location, size of organization, and other factors. The *MGMA Academic Practice Compensation and Production Survey for Faculty and Management* is an example of a report with comparative salary and productivity data for academic centers across the country. The survey breaks out data by amount of billable time, which is important because of the highly variable schedules between research, teaching, and clinical time. Salaries must also be set within the confines of the financial realities of the department or faculty plans so as not to exceed the expected total revenue, including subsidies, minus expenses. Increases in salaries should be based on understood criteria such as promotions in rank and the financial well-being of the department and organization.

Academic faculty compensation can also be determined by comparing the faculty to private practice compensation benchmarks and then basing their level of productivity and compensation to private practicing physicians. For example, if a physician produces at the 50th percentile when compared to the MGMA Physician Compensation and Production Survey for private practices or all practices, the physician receives that corresponding level of compensation (the MGMA percentile).

Salaries can also be determined by combining all the revenue sources for each physician (state funding, research support, educational base, clinical revenue, etc.) and allocating their expenses. This method requires more calculations and estimations of expected revenue and expenses and therefore is more complex to manage. Fluctuations in funding and expenses can cause volatility in compensation unless rounding or other techniques are used. One option is to set a cap on compensation. If the compensation pool exceeds the cap, the excess is set aside to fund periods of lower revenue.

Options for ensuring a minimal activity level or providing incentives for increased performance should be considered. Performance targets may be set to require a minimum number of hours in clinical or teaching activities or a minimum number of research publications or grant dollars. If targets aren't achieved, then a consequence should be defined; a potential decrease in compensation by a set amount or certain percentage can be effective options.

A more positive option is to offer a reduced base salary plus incentives. Incentives can include a share of collections or revenue for increased clinical activity or for exceeding productivity, teaching, or research goals; a share in rewards for achieving patient satisfaction targets; or some other method. The base salary can be reduced by 5–10 percent, 50 percent, or however much is agreed on to match organizational emphasis and plans. The greater a percentage that compensation is based on individual performance, the more improvement in the desired behavior will be seen. A fairly typical base compensation is around 70–80 percent of total compensation, although it is up to each organization to determine the best percentage.

The expected performance level or target to receive incentive payment needs to be set high enough or with increments to ensure continued effort toward achieving the goal but not so high as to be unattainable by most physicians or unaffordable by the organization.

Clinical Activity and Productivity Compensation

Many teaching facilities are incorporating productivity as a component in compensation as a means of dealing with the changing reimbursement and marketplace. Including at least a percentage of compensation based on productivity measures provides incentives for physicians to increase clinical activity. This increase in activity can result in increased reimbursement and number of patient encounters.

Compensation can be based on any of the productivity measures discussed in chapter 3: charges, collections, relative value units (RVUs), encounters, or patients. Using more than one measure in a plan can also help ensure physician compliance, prevent gaming the system, and will allow the department to spread incentives according to its mission.

Compensation based on work RVUs (wRVUs) or other performance measures can be implemented in any manner described in chapter 3: with a set amount of compensation per wRVU, as a percentage of total practice wRVUs, or with set incentive payments for achieving different targets in wRVUs. The latter option includes distributing an allocation from an incentive pool based on the number of RVUs over the target or the number of RVUs produced in excess of RVUs needed to cover the base salary. If a compensation per wRVU value is selected, it should be evaluated annually to ensure it is still in line with the marketplace and the organization's financial status.

Academic practices must balance the productivity incentive based on clinical activities with the other missions of the organization: teaching and research. Therefore, clinical productivity may never be as large a percentage of total compensation as in private practices but should be large enough to "gain the physicians' attention" – to provide enough incentive to encourage more clinical activity. Each department, faculty plan, or facility will have to decide what the correct percentage is for its plan. Faculties that devote 50 percent or more to research time may be asked to raise revenue through research funding to counter the decreased billable time.

Teaching and Research Recognition

Incorporating incentives for teaching and research can be more difficult than for clinical activities because there is less direct connection to a dollar value, both include a variety of activities that involve different work efforts and rewards, and it is difficult to gauge and rate the actual performance of the physician in the effort. Although there has always been a push from teaching facilities to encourage research activities and grant funding, the emphasis is increasing and is reflected in compensation formulas.

Academic medical practices have arrived at various solutions to include teaching and research in compensation formulas. One method is for department chairs or others to rate physicians on the quantity and quality of their teaching and research efforts. This subjective method is open to concerns about favoritism and must be used carefully.

A more objective method is to track the amount of teaching and research activity. Administrators track the number of teaching hours, courses, research grants, dollars in grant funding, and so on, and rank the physicians accordingly. Compensation is then based on total number of points or comparison rank with other physicians in the department or rank. Scores on student or peer surveys can also be incorporated in physician ranking.

Some academic centers have developed complex point systems to measure physician effort in various activities. Under this system, administrators and physicians record their activities, and then values or points are attributed to the activities. The two most common techniques are:

1. Assign each activity an RVU value and add the academic RVUs to the clinical RVUs; and

2. Assign each activity a point value, and calculate compensation based on total points.

For both options, the faculty or compensation committee members need to generate a list of activities in both areas. For example, under research, the list might include publication in a journal or magazine, publication in a peer-reviewed journal, co-authoring a publication, authoring or co-authoring a book, journal editing, number of grants received of X-dollar amounts, serving as principal investigator on a clinical trial, and so forth. Under teaching will be listed curriculum design; number of courses taught; number of grand rounds, lectures, or presentations; hours in student or residency supervision; and others. The list can include other factors such as committee participation, community services, completion of records and evaluations, awards and honors, and so on. The lists can be as detailed as the faculty wishes them to be, but the more detailed they are, the more accurate the data gathering and recognition will be. See Exhibits 9.1 and 9.2 for examples of faculty activities.

The most difficult step is assigning an RVU value or a point system to each activity. Values can be based on the relative number of hours and effort to complete that activity, the amount of revenue or recognition received from external sources for the activity, or the value that the organization wishes to place on the activity. The latter allows some flexibility in the system for adjusting point value depending on organizational goals and mission. For example, an initial emphasis on increasing research and grant funding may lead to higher point values for the number of grants received. It should be recognized that the point system will not be set in stone but remain

EXHIBIT 9.1　■　Faculty Reporting Form Example

The following is a subset of the schedule developed to list nonclinical activities and provide a conversion value. This practice used a point system based on estimated number of hours for each activity converted to RVUs.

Conversion Factor: 1 RH (Research Hour) = 1 EH (Education Hour) = 3 RVUs

Recording and Conversion Schedule for an Academic Surgical Practice

Activity	Self-Report Required	Verification	Measure
Grants accepted and funded $10,000–$49,000	No	Administrator	50 RH
Grants accepted and funded >$200,000	No	Administrator	300 RH
Grant written and submitted, not funded	Yes	Administrator or chairperson	15 RH/grant
Research papers – first author or corresponding author	Yes	Administrator or chairperson	30 RH/occurrence
CME presentation (regional or national)	Yes	Administrator or chairperson	5 EH/occurrence
Grand rounds or conference presentation	Yes	Administrator, head & vice chair	1 EH/occurrence
Mock orals examiner	Yes	Residency director	8 EH/occurrence
Precept medical students patient-based assessments	Yes	Clerkship director	3 EH/occurrence
Timely completion (by due date) of student and resident evaluations	Yes	Program directors	Penalize 3 EH/failure
Attendance at department faculty meetings	Yes	Swipe card	Attendance > 50% or penalize 10 EH
Structured medical student education curriculum	Yes	Clerkship director	2 EH/hour engagement

Source: Sally Rodgers, FACMPE, "Restructuring Physician Compensation in an Academic Medical Setting," ACMPE Fellowship Paper, October 2009 https://www.mgma.com/workarea/mgma_downloadasset.aspx?id=34345 (accessed February 11, 2013).

EXHIBIT 9.2 ■ Faculty Self-Assessment Form

The following is a subset of the spreadsheet used to track faculty activity in a reporting period.

Name: _____

Section: _____

TEACHING ACTIVITIES

Activity Description	Unit Value	Units	Total
Course Director (Medical School Course)	100		
Course Director (CME Course)	40		
Medical Student Lectures	10		
Mentoring of Graduate Students *List graduate students.*	6		
Extra-Departmental Lectures	6		
CME Lectures	10		
Teacher of the Year Award	100		
Total Teaching			

PUBLICATIONS AND PRESENTATIONS
Include only papers published or anticipated to be published during the measurement period.

Refereed Journal – First Author	100		
Refereed Journal – Co-Author	40		
Non-Refereed Journal – Mentor for Medical/ Graduate Students or Resident	40		
Book Chapter – First Author	60		
Case Report – Mentor for Fellow	16		
Service for Journal – Editorial Board Member	20		
National Meeting Presentations – First Author	40		
Total Publications			

GRANTS

Salary Funded via Extramural Grants *List grant name, number, % of salary covered, and your total salary for each grant. Points awarded are 0.03 per dollar of salary covered.*	0.03		
Co-Investigator – Major Grant Proposal Submitted *4 points per 1% effort or 40 points, whichever is greater*	4		
Principal Investigator – Major Grant Awarded *>$100,000 total support*	200		
Principal Investigator – Minor Grant Awarded, <$100,000	100		
Co-Investigator – Major Grant Awarded *2 points per 1% effort or 20 points, whichever is greater*	2		
Patents Awarded	100		
Total Grants			

Exhibit continued next page

EXHIBIT 9.2 ■ Faculty Self-Assessment Form (continued)

ADMINISTRATION

Note: Only claim points for administrative roles that are not associated with outside salary support.

Activity Description	Unit Value	Units	Total
Director, Medical Student Research Program	40		
Major Facility Medical Director	130		
Minor Facility Medical Director	20		
Director, Nonaccredited Fellowship Program	20		
Member, Clinical Practice Corporation Committee	16		
Chair, Department Committees	100		
Member, Department Committees	16		
Total Administration			
TOTAL SCHOLARLY/ADMINISTRATIVE ACTIVITY POINTS			

Source: Adapted from Carl R. Whittenburg, FACMPE, "Creating a Compensation Plan for an Academic Radiology Department," ACMPE Fellowship Paper, October 2011.

flexible and allow for corrections in the initial assignment of points and as changes occur in the organization or marketplace.

The teaching and research activity is gathered for each physician through a combination of department- or administration-recorded data and physicians' self-reporting. Forms should be developed to allow physicians to record the number and amount of activity not recorded by administration. Exhibits 9.1 and 9.2 are examples for subsets of faculty reporting forms and point systems developed by two academic departments.

Administrators should audit these forms to ensure that those who input the data are not gaming the system and there is fair and accurate gathering of information. Administrators should also be concerned about the complexity of developing and managing these systems, including the potential need to hire someone to track the information and audit the forms.

However, physicians may prefer this method as an accurate means of tracking and recognizing all of their activity. Another advantage of this system is the additional incentive for physicians to complete these forms since compensation or incentive payments are tied to the data, increasing the reporting of all the faculty activity. Where possible, departments should look to automate forms to allow for standardization and ease of reporting. Administration can use the data to compile and compare its faculty with other institutions and use the information to report to state funding agencies and grant sources.

Administrative, Quality, and Other Factors

Faculty compensation plans need to consider other potential components in determining compensation or incentives the same as in private practice compensation formulas. Recognition of time spent in administrative functions might be a goal of the compensation committee and the plan to encourage participation in practice committees, meetings, and leadership activities such as residency director. Department chairs, assistant or vice chairs, and other leadership positions may be provided with compensation separate from the compensation system of other faculty members. If not, recognizing the time devoted to administrative activities for these positions and others should be recognized. Chapter 5 describes various options to include compensation or incentives as part of the compensation plan.

Academic medical practices have not yet been widely impacted by value-based reimbursement, although a few have chosen to participate in demonstration programs. As this method of reimbursement spreads, organizations need to recognize the value of incorporating value-based incentives such as patient experience, quality metrics, and outcome measures. Implementing these components in compensation can be done similar to that discussed for private practices in chapter 4 and based on experiences of faculty members that have led the way.

Compensation and Incentive Pool

Faculty practices face the same issue as private practices in deciding how to fund the compensation and incentive pool. Reimbursement from clinical activity may be combined with state funding to create the compensation pool. Grant funding will either pass through directly to the faculty minus a "tax" to support department and AMC administrative functions or the funding will go to a central fund for later distribution to the physicians (minus contributions to overhead).

The incentive pool is usually created by withholding a portion of the compensation pool equal to the percentage of compensation that is equal to physician performance incentives. The center may seek additional funds to support faculty incentives including payers' incentive payments or grants. Incentives to reward clinical activity may increase reimbursement enough to cover the cost of incentive compensation. If the incentive pool fluctuates depending on the practice's income and expenses or the campus budget, then physicians will be linked to the financial performance of the organization via the amount in their incentive payments.

Structuring Incentive Compensation

Several options are available for including clinical and nonclinical activity within the incentive system. Clinical activity compensation may be considered separate from the nonclinical incentives or the incentive compensation pool can include incentives for all the activities. Either option can be structured to provide flexibility in weighting

EXHIBIT 9.3 ■ Separate Incentive Pools

Base salary	$100,000
Potential productivity-based compensation	$50,000
Teaching and research potential compensation	$50,000
Potential total compensation	$200,000

EXHIBIT 9.4 ■ Combined Incentive Pool

Base salary	$100,000
Incentive compensation pool	$100,000
Clinical productivity	40% = $40,000 potential
Teaching and research	50% = $50,000 potential
Value-based factors	10% = $10,000
Potential total compensation	$200,000

the three main missions of academic centers by shifting the percentage of compensation based on clinical services, teaching, research, and administrative functions. Exhibits 9.3 and 9.4 are examples of how the two options could be structured.

Determination of actual dollar amounts for incentive payments will be based on the method for tracking the activity measures. If an RVU-based system is used, then a dollar amount per RVU is determined and each physician's total RVUs (clinical wRVUs plus research and teaching RVUs) are multiplied by the compensation/RVU value to determine the incentive payment. Point systems can be assigned dollar values per point or points can be totaled and each physician's points determined as a percentage of the total department or faculty plan points. The incentive pool is distributed by percentage of points. One practice using an RVU system divided the total incentive or merit pool into a clinical pool and a scholarly activity pool. Each pool was divided by the total RVUs for the two activities to arrive at an RVU value. The physicians' individual RVU totals were multiplied by this value to determine their incentive or merit payment for clinical and nonclinical activities.[2]

Plan Implementation and Review

The compensation committee should proceed with plan development similar to the process described in chapter 7 for private practices but with the exception of needing to work closely with the central leadership of the faculty plan or AMC. The committee should ensure that the developing plan meets the organizational guidelines prior to releasing a completed plan.

Implementing the new compensation formula should follow the same considerations as for private practices, including testing the formula with different variables and over time to ensure that it complies with expectations and that the impact of unforeseen consequences is limited. Leadership should hold individual meetings with physicians to explain the terms and impact of the new compensation plan. Individual letters should compare faculty members' current and expected productivity data and potential changes in compensation.

Developing a physician performance report or scorecard will enable physicians to compare their productivity and nonclinical activity levels with other physicians within the AMC and with external benchmarks. The report can include wRVUs, charges, collections, summary of research and teaching activity, quality metrics, patient satisfaction scores, or other factors.

During a transition period, faculty may receive a guaranteed minimum compensation, to provide time to adjust, before completing the transition. During this period, physicians performing above previous levels or performance targets could be eligible for incentive payments.

A plan review should be conducted six months to one year after implementation, depending on the ease with which it was implemented. The review should address several questions including:

- Are physicians satisfied with the plan?

- Is the system equitable?

- Is total compensation matching expectations?

- Are the measures for rewarding clinical and nonclinical performance fair and transparent?

- Is the list of teaching and research activities comprehensive or should additional activities be included?

- Are faculty physicians and administration satisfied with the assigned values for the activities?

- Are the goals and objectives of the plan and the organization being met? If not, is it due to changing environmental factors or internal factors? Should incentives be increased or modified to obtain desired behavior?

- What have been the consequences of the plan's implementation? Are there bad, unforeseen consequences that need to be addressed?

Academic Practice Case Studies

University of Texas Southwestern Medical Center, Department of Surgery[3]

The university's leadership recognized that changes needed to be made in the faculty compensation plan to meet the challenges of declining revenue compared to costs and to prepare for changes in healthcare reimbursement. The center's administration developed a compensation plan foundation to encourage clinical productivity and included incentives of no more than 25 percent of the annual salary. The previous compensation plans varied by clinical department but were mainly salary based, and physicians received a standard increase of 2 to 3 percent each year across the board based on administrative discretion.

Physician wRVUs and compensation were compared with MGMA data to determine if compensation was in line with benchmark productivity. Implementation of the plan began with letters to each physician comparing their current and expected productivity and salary data. If current salary was at X percent of MGMA compensation, then the physician was expected to have wRVUs at the same or greater percentile. The current salary was continued through the first year with physicians able to earn additional compensation for higher productivity but no decreases for lower productivity. After implementation, the administration could approve a salary decrease for lower productivity.

The departments were allowed by administration to develop the details of the incentive plans to match their specialty and culture. The department's compensation committee included the department chair and chairs from each division, the department administrator, and the financial affairs manager. Division chairs provided the contact with faculty and coordinated the selection of group incentive metrics. Some divisions used monthly meetings to relay information on plan development; others used individual meetings or other communication means.

The incentive compensation is based on two components. The first component is based on the faculty member exceeding the number of wRVUs expected of them. The second component is based on two to three metrics chosen by faculty with all divisions choosing a mixture of individual and group metrics. Examples include: completing and closing patient records in a timely manner, operating room infection control, patient satisfaction, and quality metrics. University administration reviewed and approved the final incentive plans.

Faculty members will be eligible for the incentive compensation only after achieving the performance targets – they are not prorated. The two to three metrics are equally weighted in determining compensation.

Promotions in rank are rewarded with an average 10 percent increase, independent of productivity. Faculty members with 50 percent or greater research time are expected to raise additional revenue dollars through increased research grants. New physicians are subsidized up to four or five years to develop a research base and sufficient grant funding.

Physicians serving in administrative roles or positions receive additional income paid biannually for their time and effort. The additional income is specific to the roles and varies depending on the role and amount of time involved.

Shirley Zwinggi, administrator, and Steven Samuel, financial affairs manager, both participated in the development of the compensation plans in the department. They believe it is important to have both an administrator and a financial manager present to provide the financial explanation and reports as well as information from the administrative side to explain the reasoning for the new plans and how the plans will be implemented.

Academic Radiology Department[4]

The department realized that the previous compensation system created inequities since compensation was based on negotiations during hiring rather than an objective measure. The faculty was also focused primarily on clinical rather than teaching and research activities. A new chair began the process to develop a new plan that was more transparent and equitable, and recognized clinical and scholarly efforts.

A committee was formed of the department chair, the department business administrator, and five physician members elected by the entire faculty. The committee reviewed literature on the topic, compensation and productivity benchmark reports, and information on the plan the chair had introduced at a previous location. Work RVUs were selected to measure physicians' clinical activity, but the RVU system was modified to provide greater value for plain radiographs which had low RVU value than for computed tomography (CT) and other imaging services. The concern was that physicians would avoid lower-value services or would overutilize other services.

The committee developed a faculty assessment form (FAF) to track teaching, publications and presentations, grants and other research, and administrative activities. The list is extensive with teaching having 11 items; publications and presentations, 39 items; grants, 14 items; and administration, 29 items. Section chiefs reviewed the FAF prior to sharing it with faculty who were asked to provide feedback after completing a sample of the form. Each item is assigned an RVU value, called an academic RVU. A condensed version of the form is included as Exhibit 9.2.

The committee settled on a risk pool of 5 percent, evenly divided between clinical and scholarly activity. Because of concerns about drastic changes in compensation under the new plan, the amount that compensation could change the first year was capped at a 5 percent increase or decrease.

Under the new plan, compensation includes a salary based on a minimum salary determined by benchmark comparison, administrative leadership compensation, academic rank, and length of time with the institution. In addition, faculty members are eligible for merit compensation of up to 5 percent. Merit compensation is determined by dividing the total dollar amount of the category (clinical or scholarly) by the total RVUs in that area. For example:

- Clinical merit pool = $500,000

- Clinical RVU production = 100,000

- Clinical merit pool divided by clinical RVU production

- ($500,000 / 100,000) = $5 per RVU

The department recognized the value of several steps in the process of developing and implementing a successful compensation formula:

- Selection of committee members by the faculty enabled faculty buy-in and recognition of potential issues before the plan was released;

- Transparency during the process was vital in gaining early approval of the plan;

- Recognizing clinical activity did not increase clinical numbers due to the nature of radiology;

- Incentives for scholarly activity would increase physician efforts. This was shown to be true with a 25 percent increase in publications and 81 percent increase in points related to grants in the second year after implementation.

- The importance of reviewing the FAF and the plan after implementation to ensure that it adequately captures and encourages appropriate efforts.

The success in the plan's effort to increase teaching, research, and administrative activities led to an increase in the merit pool to 20 percent to encourage additional effort. Not only have academic activities increased, but faculty members are now volunteering to serve in administrative functions. The merit pool remains evenly divided between clinical and nonclinical activity.

MetroHealth Medical Center, Cleveland, Ohio[5]

MetroHealth's Emergency Department is a Level 1 trauma center and the largest Medicaid provider in the state. Its physicians supervise an emergency medicine residency program. Several issues were recognized, including the need to increase volume, improve access, and improve customer service. A series of changes were implemented, including development and implementation of a new physician incentive program.

At the time, faculty members were employed on salary-based compensation plans with only 1 to 2 percent incentive for quality and documentation goals.

A consultant was hired to review physician compensation and help in designing an incentive program. An incentive compensation committee was formed and charged with "making recommendations about the design of the incentive program." Results were reviewed by the department chair and modified by senior administration.

The new plan had three goals:

1. Maintain the base salary since physicians were worried that incentive payments would be from a reduction in base compensation.

2. Incentives should not be a high percentage of total pay since commitments to teaching, research, and administrative responsibilities needed to continue.

3. The plan must be easy to understand "with identified pathways for performance improvement and measurable goals" and simple to administer with currently available data.

The result was RVU based but included quality, patient satisfaction, and academic performance components. The incentive pool was initially funded by an increase in RVUs and capped at 10 percent of total base salaries. Allocation was based on RVUs over the median in an MGMA academic survey.

The compensation formula consisted of:

- 15 percent for academic performance based on points for different activities. For example, daily 10-minute lectures = 1 point, article publication = 150 points, and Teacher of the Year award = 100 points;

- 5 percent for department goals for administrative, quality, and patient satisfaction goals. For example, reducing the number of patients who left before evaluation, meeting median scores in patient satisfaction, meeting or exceeding budget goals; and

- 5 percent for the chair's discretion to recognize other administrative activities.

After implementation, improvements that were tracked included: 8 percent increase in average number of patients/hour, 17 percent increase in RVU production, and patients who left before being seen dropped to 2 percent. It was determined that each dollar in bonus payment resulted in a $6 increase in revenue.

End Notes

1. Sally Rodgers, "Restructuring Physician Compensation in an Academic Medical Setting," ACMPE Fellowship Paper (October 2009), https://www.mgma.com/workarea/mgma_downloadasset.aspx?id=34345 (accessed February 11, 2013).

2. Carl R. Whittenburg, FACMPE, "Creating a Compensation Plan for an Academic Radiology Department," ACMPE Fellow Paper (October 2011), http://www.mgma.com/workarea/downloadasset.aspx?id=1368298 (accessed April 15, 2013).

3. Shirley Zwinggi, administrator, and Steven Samuel, financial affairs manager, University of Texas Southwestern Medical Center, Department of Surgery, Dallas, Texas, interview with author, February 12, 2013.

4. See note 2 above (accessed February 27, 2013).

5. Charles L. Emerman, MD, Jonathan Siff, MD, and Alfred F. Connors Jr., MD, "Hospital Reaps Rewards from RVU Incentive-Based Program," *MGMA Connexion* (November/December 2010), https://www.mgma.com/workarea/mgma_downloadasset.aspx?id=40204 (accessed February 26, 2013).

CHAPTER 10

Putting It All Together: Examples in Compensation Planning

As stated in chapter 4, value-based factors may be the most challenging issue to incorporate in physician compensation formulas since they are more difficult to track and implement than collections or relative value units (RVUs). Implementation of value-based factors also requires a paradigm shift in how medical practices operate and providers interact with patients. Physicians are now more accountable for adhering to protocols and recommended processes. More emphasis is being placed on patient interactions, including patients' involvement in their care and changing behavior to improve their health.

Because of these challenges in the new environment, it is helpful to look at case studies of health organizations that are making the transition and incorporating value-based factors as part of their physician compensation methodology.

Simple Compensation Methodologies

Equal Share Distribution[1]

A pulmonary practice in Nevada succeeded under an equal share compensation method. Equal distribution of the compensation pool (revenue minus expenses) worked well for several reasons:

- Physicians' schedules are equally distributed between the hospital, office, and the practice's sleep center;

- Because of the nature of pulmonary medicine, there is little control on whether patients are seen in the office or hospital: whoever is on schedule sees the patients that present at that time;

- Equal activity and schedules means equal share of expenses; and

- The practice is the only pulmonary practice in the community, so there isn't any competition or fight for patients in the marketplace.

Physicians working part-time schedules receive a proportionate decrease in their share. The group participates in a Physician Quality Reporting System (PQRS), and the incentive payments are entered in the general fund for distribution as part of the total compensation pool since success under the PQRS is seen as an organizational effort. The practice implemented disincentives for incorrect documentation with a potential decrease in a physician's share of compensation but has not had to enforce this policy.

Practice leadership is recognized through a monthly stipend, including pay for the CEO, board officers, and medical director of the sleep lab. Donna Knapp, MGMA healthcare consultant, who served as administrator of the pulmonary practice for many years, believes that financial incentives for practice citizenship are a valuable tool. "It lessens the pain of nonclinical activities," she states, and encourages participation especially for those who are good at leadership.

Salary Plus Incentive

This section provides three examples of medical practices that implemented compensation methodologies based on salary plus incentives.

Three-Physician Practice[2]

The first compensation plan was straight salary, but salaries were above the regional norm and not reflective of declining reimbursement in an economic downturn. The practice administrator "knew that the model had to align with the practice goals and the patients' best interests." The goal was to develop a plan that was fair, rewarded physicians in proportion to their effort, balanced risk and reward, and was simple enough to be easy to implement and understand. The plan also needed goals that were attainable and realistic.

The administrator considered several models and presented three options to the physicians to elicit their feedback: equal shares distribution, productivity, and salary plus incentive. Other options were not presented because they didn't match the practice culture or climate. Salary plus incentive was agreed as the best option, but physicians couldn't agree on how to determine incentive pay – seniority, charges, or revenue. Each physician would benefit most from one option but were concerned about the other two options. When disagreement continued after several meetings, the administrator offered a solution.

The administrator decided on a plan based on budgeted net revenue for practice divided by several factors:

- 5 percent would be set aside for a reserve fund;
- 75 percent would be used for salaries divided equally among physicians;
- 10 percent divided by seniority based on a percentage of each physician's number of years in the practice; and
- 10 percent based on productivity calculated by the percentage of total RVUs each physician had generated the previous year.

Since the plan resulted in a decrease in compensation due to a decrease in practice revenue, physicians were not happy with the plan. The administrator brought in the practice accountant to explain the practice's financial picture. Physicians finally agreed to the proposed plan and grew to appreciate it. The administrator realized that the accountant should have been brought in sooner since his objective view was needed to make physicians realize the true financial picture.

The advice offered based on this practice's experience is: "Keep it simple. Like employees, physicians need to have measurable, attainable goals. They need to be able to focus on their job, not a complicated compensation model."

Family Practice Group[3]

This group debated the advantages and disadvantages of several models and settled on a salary plus bonus/incentive. They identified the following benefits of this model:

- Supports team environment by decreasing competitiveness;
- Includes a known amount as the base, reducing risk for the physicians while maintaining financial stability of the practice;
- Incentivizes and rewards behaviors and efforts the group wishes to promote; and
- Flexible to adjust to changes in revenue, activities, data analysis capabilities, and so forth.

The salary was set at 75 percent of the previous year's mean/median earnings, but to receive the full salary, physicians must work at least 90 percent of a full-time-equivalent (FTE) schedule and 90 percent of the productivity measure. The practice chose number of office visits and share of call coverage as the productivity measures. If targets are not reached, then the salary is reduced by a calculated amount.

The incentive payment was based on group and individual efforts divided equally between two pools:

1. Site incentive pool, which was divided equally among partners/shareholders; and

2. Individual incentive pool, which includes several factors that are currently measurable and assigned a percentage of the incentive pool:

   - **Special qualifications**, 5 percent, meant to reward for obstetric and nursing home services and community physicals.

   - **Productivity**, 20 percent, based on percentage of patient encounters;

   - **Citizenship**, 10 percent, to factor in "individual effort and good behavior;"

   - **Panel size**, 20 percent;

   - **Resource utilization**, 10 percent, includes physician's rate of referrals, imaging, and so on, compared with the group's mean;

   - **Seniority**, 5 percent, each physician will receive a portion of this money based on his or her years in practice within the group; and

   - **Overhead/cost control**, 30 percent, calculated by determining overhead costs per physician (direct expenses and share of indirect variable costs) and dividing by the average for the practice. Distribution is based on equal share plus or minus a percentage point for each point above or below the average.

The group included administrative functions as set stipends added to the practice's fixed overhead costs. The group planned to include quality and patient satisfaction as soon as they were confident of the data for these measures. The measures and percentages will be reviewed regularly to ensure they reflect the group's goals.

Base Salary with Tiered RVU Incentive[4]

One hospital employed eight primary care physicians (PCPs) under different contracts with different compensation models. The models were inconsistent and did not motivate the physicians because the goals were difficult to achieve and not clearly understood. The hospital realized the need to implement a new compensation plan with clear and consistent metrics and hired a consulting team to assist in plan development. A work group was formed consisting of the consultants, physicians, and members of the administrative team. The committee identified three options:

1. Work RVU (wRVU) based plan;

2. Revenue minus expenses plus subsidy to achieve a guaranteed level of compensation; or

3. Do nothing.

The first option was selected by the physicians, and administration agreed. Physicians would continue to receive a guaranteed salary but with the option of earning additional compensation based on their productivity. A tiered plan was developed as follows:

- **Tier I:** Work RVUs up to the 40th MGMA percentile are compensated at the median MGMA compensation per wRVU value;

- **Tier II:** In addition to Tier I compensation, wRVUs between the 40th percentile and the 75th percentile are compensated at the 75th percentile value for compensation per wRVU; and

- **Tier III:** In addition to Tiers I and II, all wRVUs greater than the 75th percentile are compensated at the 90th percentile.

Productivity-based compensation calculated following the above method would be compared to the base salary. If the former exceeds the base salary, the difference is paid as incentive compensation.

The administrator developed a new physician report that clearly detailed expected and achieved performance, including encounters and wRVUs by setting. The administrator met individually with physicians on a monthly basis to review the reports and answer questions. A three-month period was used to prepare the practice prior to implementing the new plan.

Since physicians were involved in the plan selection, they believed it was fair and increased their trust in the administration.

More Complex Methodologies

The following case studies share the challenges that have been faced as these healthcare organizations have transitioned to compensation methodologies that are more complex.

Productivity Plus Incentive

Billings Clinic[5]

Based in Billings, Mont., the Billings Clinic is a community-owned healthcare organization consisting of a multispecialty physician group practice, a hospital, and a skilled nursing and assisted living facility. The productivity-based compensation system is determined by RVUs. The incentive system uses a set dollar amount for some physicians while others have 3 percent withheld for quality incentives. Some specialties compensation formulas include value-based measures that are also considered core quality issues, including reducing hospital readmission, blood usage, and length of stay. The Quality, Service, Leadership (QSL) incentive program affects 5–10 percent of the incentive compensation. Specialty-specific metrics include core measures and compliance with condition-specific guidelines or protocols.

Lexington Clinic[6]

Productivity-based compensation plans are the norm for the more than 150 physicians in multispecialty Lexington Clinic in Kentucky. RVUs were chosen as the productivity measure since it is payer blind. Direct expenses are allocated to each physician, including a share of rent, support staff salaries and benefits, equipment, phones, and computers. Indirect expenses are allocated by a share based on physician revenue. Compensation is the physician's net revenue minus direct expenses. New physicians are on guaranteed salaries for two years, determined by industry survey data.

A quarterly "citizenship bonus" is used to encourage physician participation in committees, educational presentations, completion of records and billing, practice leadership positions, and so on. Each activity is assigned a number of points, and points have a set value of $312.50. The total bonus amount available per physician is $2,500 per quarter.

Complex Methodology with Value-Based Incentives

CoxHealth, Springfield, Mo.[7]

CoxHealth began shifting toward a pay-for-performance (P4P) compensation plan not because they were receiving P4P payments but because of the general trend toward alignment and integration as part of an overall health system improvement. Commercial payers are not yet paying under P4P programs, but there have been discussions, and CoxHealth recently joined one of Medicare's bundled payment programs. The integrated system is moving toward a managed, coordinated care approach that must be supported throughout the organization. David Taylor, vice president, Regional Services, believes the evolving compensation plans support the culture and philosophy, and align physicians with the organization's mission, vision, and values:

> CoxHealth's mission is to improve the health of the communities we serve through quality health care, education and research. Our vision is to be the best for those who need us. We value safety, compassion, respect and integrity.

CoxHealth's employed physician group is comprised of more than 230 providers located in more than 60 clinics. Each specialty has a defined compensation plan with about half of the physicians on an incentive-based compensation formula. Currently, the medical group leadership develops models or basic concepts using MGMA data to benchmark. They work with physicians in each group to identify goals and then negotiate the plan details. For example, when hospitalists requested a shift to a wRVU system, a plan was established and negotiated with the physicians.

CoxHealth has implemented a Physician Compensation Committee to provide legal and compliance oversight plus consistency across the system. Members include physicians, health system leadership, attorneys, and the compliance officer. Currently, CoxHealth uses three basic compensation methods:

1. Fixed pay or salary;

2. Traditional collections minus expenses; and

3. Work RVU-based compensation.

The salary or fixed-pay method is a small percentage of physicians, usually hospital based. This includes subspecialists, such as pediatric subspecialists, for which there is an identified need for that specialty but not enough demand to support a productivity-based formula. Physicians on salary are expected to meet productivity expectations, and a small percentage of compensation is available in a P4P bonus payment.

The traditional collections-minus-expenses plans are used to mirror physicians in private practice. It is used for PCPs and many surgical specialties. The formula provides productivity incentive but also accountability toward expenses. P4P incentives are being considered to include in the plans. The wRVU-based methodology is reserved for a few physicians, including hospitalists. Since they have less control over payer mix and which patients they see, the physicians believed it was a more accurate measure than collections.

P4P elements are built into plans or considered for plans and will generally represent 5 to 8 percent of compensation. Nationally, there are discussions that P4P should represent 20 to 30 percent of physician compensation. CoxHealth is tracking this and will modify their plans accordingly. Different measures are used depending on payer incentives and practice specifics. Measures are also selected based on ease of tracking and reporting. There have been issues when the hospital structure has changed the reporting system and methodology, which impacts the data reporting for physician performance. Several quality measures are based on HEDIS (Healthcare Effectiveness Data and Information Set) scores, such as percentage of diabetics receiving eye exams and the percentage of patients over 50 having colonoscopy or other cancer screenings.

P4P and bonuses are dependent on other measures, including patient satisfaction, record completion, continuing medical education program development, or meeting attendance. Some measures require achieving the full target to receive a bonus, no partial bonus payments, while others will pay out for improvement from previous reports. For example, physicians must attend 75–80 percent of hospital, committee, or specialty meetings to receive a bonus, and if 100 percent of meetings are attended, they receive extra. The P4P compensation is funded through a two- to three-dollar withhold for each wRVU. Physicians know their status related to the bonus program through the physician performance report (Exhibit 10.1), which states the indicator,

EXHIBIT 10.1 ■ CoxHealth Physician Performance Report 2012

Clinic:

Physician: 2012

		2012
	Total RVUs	—

#	% of Total P4P Bonus $	RVU Value	Indicator	Score					Total Physician Payout
1	0%	$ —	Patient Satisfaction						
				Physician Actual Percentile	Physician Net Change Percentile	% Payout Actual	% Payout Net Change		
				0	0	0%	0%		$ —

Methodology:

1. _____

2. _____

3. _____

#	% of Total Bonus $	RVU Value	Indicator	Physician Attendance Rate	Percent Payout	Total Physician Payout
2	0%	$ —	Meeting Attendance			$ —

Methodology:

1. _____

2. _____

3. _____

#	% of Total Bonus $	Maximum Value/RVU	Indicator	#	Percent Payout	Annual Total Physician Payout
3	0%	$ —	Record Documentation 1	0	0%	$ —

Methodology:

1. _____

2. _____

3. _____

#	% of Total Bonus $	Maximum Value/RVU	Indicator	% of Charts with Problems Documented	Percent Payout	Annual Total Physician Payout
4	0%	$ —	Record Documentation 2	0%	0%	$ —

Methodology:

1. _____

2. _____

3. _____

		Total Payout	$ —

Source: David Taylor, vice president, Regional Services (Integrated Physicians Group), CoxHealth. Used with permission.

indicator's weighting, physician's ranking, and the amount of compensation related to the factor.

Future changes being considered in compensation and incentive programs are incentives for care management, reducing readmissions, and other utilization management factors. Data from the health plan are being analyzed to consider including factors on panel size, patient risk level, care team participation or supervision, and shared savings options.

Primary Care and Value-Based Emphasis[8–10]

Physicians at Dean Clinic in Madison, Wis., a physician-owned clinic and part of the integrated Dean Health System, saw the need to shift from compensating physicians based on volume to paying for quality. In 2009, Dean Clinic and health plan leaders realized that PCPs influence 80 percent of the total patient care costs but were receiving compensation equal to only 6 percent of the total cost. The organization decided to implement a primary care redesign toward a model of emphasizing wellness and maintenance of health along with maximizing the patient experience. Dean Clinic introduced the medical home model and shifted to value-based compensation for PCPs.

The previous model was nearly 100 percent based on productivity. Over several years, the productivity-based percentage of compensation decreased and nonproductivity incentives increased. The group started with tracking and benchmarking nonproductivity measures before incorporating them into the compensation formula. By 2012, the compensation formula paid at 115% of market compensation with 60 percent determined by productivity, 20 percent based on population management metrics, and 35 percent by value-based measures including quality, efficiency, patient satisfaction, and use of technology. Under the new compensation formula, physicians were able to earn similar compensation as before or even an increased amount. Craig E. Samitt, MD, MBA, president and CEO of Dean Health System, explains: "We set the initial incentives to a very small percentage and we made the goals achievable; once the physicians saw that they could reach their goals and they were comfortable with the new model, then we raised the bar."

In 2013, PCPs transitioned to a formula based on the following:

- 50 percent productivity, based on RVUs;
- 30 percent panel size, adjusted for age and gender;
- 10 percent medical cost control; and
- 20 percent on service and quality.

Measures included in calculating compensation include CG-CAHPS (Clinician and Group Consumer Assessment of Healthcare Providers and Systems) satisfaction and access scores, staff evaluations of physicians, cost of care, cost efficiency, and quality metrics. Individual and group CG-CAHPS scores and budget goals were incorporated. Under this formula, physicians have the opportunity to earn 110–115 percent of market-based compensation to encourage physicians to concentrate on the incentives. "The way this is designed, it takes [physicians] off the treadmill and helps them to be more thoughtful with patients," states Samitt.

The group's leaders admit that it is "still a work in progress." Fee-for-service (FFS) reimbursement remains a factor and RVU-based compensation will continue. However, in the future, physicians may see further reduction in productivity and introduction of a base, guaranteed salary. A productivity factor may always be included to ensure that an expected level of effort continues.

Samitt offers the following lessons learned from the transformation:

- It takes a team effort. The process was led by a team of physicians and the Dean board of directors;

- "Comp re-design doesn't solve everything." It takes more than the compensation formula to change the organization. Vision, peer pressure, values, physician compacts, data, and even guilt are needed to complete the transition;

- Compensation must be balanced between a variety of factors: production, service, quality, cost, and growth;

- Individual, department, and organization-wide goals and incentives must be included;

- Offering options to receive incentives eased the transition;

- Initial incentives were set at 1–2 percent each to appear less threatening;

- Easily achievable goals were identified at first;

- As physicians become comfortable with the concept, increase the percentages, reduce the options, change the metrics, and raise the thresholds over time.

Transition to a Patient-Centered Plan: Geisinger Health System[11–13]

An integrated health services organization with a health plan based in Danville, Pa., Geisinger first implemented a compensation plan with incentives in 2001 to align with an organizational redesign to focus on patient-centered primary care and inpatient and specialty care. The redesign was implemented with the goal of "improving outcomes while reducing costs, enhancing the provider experience, and raising financial performance. The health system and group practice leaders have long believed that a quality- and value-driven incentive program is critical to reward both individual and group progress."

The compensation plan has evolved several times since 2001 with changing emphases and new healthcare delivery models. The organization recognized the importance of having "guiding principles" in place prior to beginning the compensation plan development process. The principles identify mutual goals and expectations and agree on the philosophy and framework for the future of the organization and physicians within it. A focus group developed the guiding principles through iterative process: identifying initial concepts, presenting the information, gathering comments, incorporating comments, then finalizing and presenting the final principles.

Change management techniques were important in smoothing the process and gaining buy-in. Regular communications occurred before implementing each change. Presentations were led by leadership teams and formatted to ensure a clear and consistent message. With more than 600 physicians, it was more effective to present guiding principles and draft compensation plans in small groups.

Compensation principles developed for the compensation plan were:

- Individual physicians should have the ability to impact their compensation;
- Those who contribute more will be compensated more;
- Factors other than productivity will also be rewarded;
- Factors that impact results rapidly and significantly will be rewarded first; and
- Parameters and processes will evolve as measurement tools and results improve.

Communication tools that were developed during the plan development process included:

1. A productivity report for each physician with key statistics, trends, benchmarks, and rankings to compare with a group of peers. This report was posted on the intranet on a monthly basis.

2. A personal scorecard for each six-month compensation cycle presenting results of each criterion in the compensation plan. The medical director uses the scorecard to review with physicians, discussing criteria and the impact on compensation along with expectations for the future. Scores for that physician as well as trends and comparisons are included.

The implementation process included many steps:

- Communicating the need for change and "gaining" acceptance for change;
- Developing a timeline and goals for the implementation process;

- Using limited criteria with small rewards in the initial rollout;

- Celebrating successes as steps in implementation as they were achieved;

- Constant communication and quickly addressing issues/questions that arose; and

- Increases in criteria, risk, and reward occurred over time with the possibility of avoiding penalties if physicians modified their behavior.

An organizational priority of improving patient satisfaction was the first criterion. Satisfaction scores from the previous 12 months were presented prior to compensation distribution, providing physicians the opportunity to explain and address possible exceptions. The reward began as a lump sum if a physician scored one standard deviation (SD) above the mean, and there was no penalty for below the mean. The second six-month review provided a larger reward for scores above two SDs. At the next six-month review, compensation was modified by a percentage of salary rather than a fixed amount, and nonphysician providers and support staff were included in the incentive plan. The third six-month cycle also included a penalty for unacceptable patient scores but with an option to avoid the penalty if patient communication training was completed. The program and satisfaction scores were reviewed after two years: the percentage of physicians with patient satisfaction scores more than one SD above the mean doubled from 15 to 33 percent. There was a matching decline in the number of physicians who scored less than one SD below the norm.

Later changes included adding incentives for productivity. Productivity measures are based on surveys of similar large group practices. Results after this iteration included an increase in patient satisfaction scores by 55 percentiles in 1.5 years and an 18 percent increase in FFS revenue in one year. The latter led to improved patient access and an increase in the number of new patients. Based on physician focus groups, the system changed to a quarterly reward instead of six-month payments to provide better connection with performance.

The plan in 2012 includes several differences for primary care and specialty physicians. Compensation for PCPs is 78.5 percent based on salary that is adjusted every six months based on FFS work units from the previous 12 months. Eight percent is based on participation in medical homes, and 13.5 percent is at risk/incentive payments. The 13.5 percent incentive compensation is broken down as follows:

- 60 percent for quality;

- 6 percent for citizenship; and

- 34 percent for financial performance.

Quality measures include implementing care processes for chronic disease management, increasing the number of patients using the patient portal, improved patient satisfaction scores, and various quality measures. The measures are dependent on organizational or unit quality focus areas that are identified each year, and a committee of physicians recommends adjusting the incentive program to match the change of focus.

Patient-centered medical homes (PCMHs) under the organization's ProvenHealth Navigator receive additional funds to implement and improve case management, patient transition, and data analysis to improve clinical operations. Each physician in a medical home receives an additional $1,800 per month because of the additional complexity in care management. PCMH physicians qualify for quality incentives based on the number of quality measure targets that are achieved. Money comes from a pool developed by the difference in actual cost of care versus expected cost if patients weren't enrolled in a PCMH program.

Specialty physicians' compensation is 80 percent based on productivity and efficiency compared to large group practice benchmarks. The 20 percent that is based on incentive is divided as follows:

- Quality = 40 percent;

- Innovation = 10 percent;

- Legacy, defined as contributing to leadership, education, and research = 10 percent;

- Contribution toward growth of Geisinger's market = 15 percent; and

- Financial performance as measured by RVUs during the previous six months = 25 percent.

The two productivity measures in base salary and incentive determination are intended to encourage productivity but are not so high as to encourage inappropriate levels of activities. The quality metrics, usually four to five specific measures, are chosen for each specialty and decided by specialty leaders and senior management. Specialists receive recognition for implementing programs or supporting primary care to improve overall patient health. For example, recognition for endocrinologists who developed programs carried out by many PCPs that led to exceeding goals of care for diabetic patients. Physicians are also rewarded for compliance with Geisinger's ProvenCare guidelines for episodic care management. A sample goal for innovation included developing wound service with a goal of reducing length of stay. Recognition under the legacy category included completing a certain percentage of resident evaluations within 30 days. Developing resources in Spanish led to a reward under the growth category.

The majority of Geisinger's revenue still comes from FFS maintaining the emphasis on productivity in the compensation plan. The new compensation plan resulted in an increase in clinical services revenue by 10 percent but also shifted compensation from below survey averages to above. The group also has a lower turnover rate than similar medical groups.

There are still ongoing issues related to compensation methodology, including balancing individual and unit-based incentives, encouraging teamwork and collaboration, incorporating compensation for teaching, and difficulty in including efficiency in the formula. The latter is partially addressed by the annual performance reviews, which include analysis of episode-of-care patterns.

Integrated System with 20 Percent Incentive[14]

Located in New Hampshire, Dartmouth-Hitchcock (D-H) includes a multispecialty physician group practice, an academic medical center, two hospitals, and a cancer center. The health system has 23 certified PCMH sites, and participated in the Centers for Medicare & Medicaid Services (CMS) Physician Group Practice Demonstration project and Cigna's Collaborative Accountable Care initiative. D-H currently participates in a number of accountable care organizations (ACOs).

Christine A. Schon, vice president, Community Group Practices, said the previous compensation formula had been telling physicians to "be productive but, by the way, watch out for quality." The organization realized the need to shift and include compensating for quality, not just telling physicians to watch for it.

The new incentive compensation system for PCPs includes 80 percent based on productivity and 20 percent on nonproductivity. The group wanted a large enough percentage to be a meaningful incentive. Productivity compensation is based on wRVUs and were chosen because the not-for-profit organization wanted payer-blind productivity measures. Four equally rated factors are included in the incentive determination:

1. Meaningful use adherence;

2. Patient satisfaction;

3. First quality metric; and

4. Second quality metric.

The quality metrics are chosen by each division or location. Physicians and administrators select the metrics by looking at the location's patient population or scores on quality metrics. For example, one location chose hypertension metrics and others chose diabetes.

Meaningful use was selected since most physicians are near the targets. Including a relatively easy target means physicians will see success and at least partial incentive payment early on. Patient satisfaction may also be fairly easy since most scores are high now.

The plan includes graduated incentive payments, meaning some payment received for achieving one goal or part of one goal. Providers are eligible for a potential 5 percent bonus for achieving or exceeding all four goals. No additional reimbursement is provided to the PCMH certified sites since the concept is part of the mission and core services.

Schon said the issue now is that organizations are in the middle of change in reimbursement and therefore in the middle of compensation formula changes. It's too new to incentive reimbursement to know if changes in compensation methodology will achieve the desired results. A new plan will probably be implemented by 2015 that will include measures related to efficiency and cost of care.

Quality-Adjusted RVU Method[15]

The Southeast Permanente Medical Group (TSPMG), an integrated health system based in Atlanta, Ga., chose a combination of productivity and efficiency, quality and patient satisfaction for its primary care department. Work RVUs were chosen to track productivity. HEDIS measures for diabetes and cardiovascular disease management were selected for assessing process of care and outcomes since they are well-documented and accepted measures and offer the opportunity to benchmark with external data. The third component was patient satisfaction data since it is an organizational priority to provide a superior patient experience.

The group determined its own conversion factor for each RVU based on market payments and internal budget. Quality indicators were benchmarked against other physicians in the group, so data are based on similar demographics. An index score of 1.0 is average for the department, and physicians are ranked below, at, or above average. A score of 1.0 earns physicians a payment of 34 percent of the TSPMG conversion factor for each wRVU that physicians produced. Patient satisfaction benchmarks and rewards are calculated in the same manner. The productivity and efficiency component is based on evaluation-and-management encounters, procedures, and scheduled telephone and e-visits.

Results three years after implementation included improved patient accessibility (a 360 percent increase in telephone and e-visits), increased patient satisfaction, and higher quality scores. Physician compensation has increased as well as morale and satisfaction. The health system continues to review the model to ensure that benchmark comparisons reflect its goals and the changing marketplace. A new staff position was created dedicated to the development and administration of current and new P4P models. Specialty departments also became interested in emulating the model.

ACO Examples – Incentives and Distribution of Shared Savings

The following examples provide ideas on how provider entities, including one group practice and two integrated systems, have decided to structure provider incentives and distribute any shared savings or other form of reimbursement incentives. The distribution examples provide some clues about how medical groups participating in shared savings or bundled programs could structure internal compensation formulas.

Coastal Carolina Health Care[16]

Coastal Carolina, based in New Bern, N.C., decided to form its own ACO because it believed that healthcare is changing and the practice must prepare for it, plus the physicians knew they could be successful and benefit from the incentive payments. The group decided not to affiliate with a hospital because the real change starts with PCPs, and supporting their services should lead to a reduction in hospitalizations. Stephen W. Nuckolls, CEO, is concerned that most ACOs will distribute shared savings based on which components of the entity see the greatest reduction in services (and revenue), and hospital services are the greatest expenses in patient care. He acknowledges that this puts his physicians under pressure for achieving all the savings, but they will reap all the distribution.

Coastal Carolina has more than 40 providers, two-thirds of which are primary care. The different locations and departments develop their own compensation formulas subject to board approval. The plans vary from production based to equal share or salary plus bonus. Owners are eligible for distribution of profits, including revenue from the ancillary services that the group owns.

Each physician receives a monthly scorecard showing his or her status on patient satisfaction and quality metrics. They are also able to view online the status of their patients based on treatment protocols.

Value-based metrics aren't currently included in the compensation determination because FFS is still the main source of reimbursement. Nuckolls also believes that if patients are satisfied, they will stay with the practice and recommend the practice to others, which increases revenue and physician income. The culture and mission of Coastal Carolina are aimed at providing better care and lower costs. These goals are integrated throughout the organization and with the physician scorecard. Compensation won't be based on quality and costs until the reimbursement supports the change.

The medical group does participate in PQRS and meaningful use. Nuckolls explained how the CMS payments for participation are distributed:

We treat PQRS and ePrescribe incentive payments as an additional Medicare payment that is added to each provider's cash collections. The gross amount of cash collections is then subject to overhead and run through the department pay plan. We did this partly because these payments were made by the government in lieu of inflation increases in payments.

Meaningful Use Payments are distributed directly to each doctor when received and are not part of the department pay plans for shareholder physicians. Some non-shareholders were treated differently depending on how many hours they worked and how long they had been with the organization. Each department ultimately made this decision.

We treated these payments this way for the following reasons: (1) The cost of implementing and purchasing our EHR had taken place in earlier periods, (2) The program paying these amounts was truly an additional program, and (3) We felt it important to our culture to not dictate to our providers that they had to use the technology in a particular way; therefore, we could say "you don't have to use the EHR in this way but you will not get your bonus if you don't." All physicians ultimately came to the conclusion that it was in the best financial interest to make the workflow changes and they have all received payments.

The initial shared savings payment the group receives will be allocated to fund the infrastructure needed to implement the ACO and future program expenses. Nuckolls is developing a formula for distributing shared savings payments that will go toward incentivizing physicians to help achieve the goals. Four main factors will be used for determining each physician's share of the distribution:

1. Equal distribution to support and acknowledge the team effort in achieving goals and shared savings.

2. Panel size of Medicare patients adjusted for average risk of patient. The group relies on Medicare's HCC-RAF (Hierarchical Condition Category–Risk Adjustment Factor) scores in determining risk adjustment.

3. Resource utilization calculated as average cost per patient or actual costs for total patient panel. This component will be based on costs that physicians have more control of, including number of tests and imaging, hospitalization rate per thousand population, number of readmissions, and emergency department utilization. If the panel size is small enough to be impacted by a small percentage of patients with extremely high costs of care or unexpected episodes, these outliers may be removed from the calculation. Physicians with above-expected costs would not receive payment for this factor.

4. ACO quality metrics. Physician's scores will be compared with peers in the practice and the CMS data.

Nuckolls offers the following viewpoint about ACOs:

> *The incentive of an ACO is to take people with bad behavior and try to change that behavior. Taking non-compliant patients and turning them around by offering the right care is the right thing to do for the patient and brings a profit to the ACO.*

ProHealth Solutions, Wisconsin[17]

The ProHealth Care hospital system of Waukesha, Wis., and the Waukesha Elmbrook Health Care (WEHC) independent practice association (IPA) united to form the ProHealth Solutions ACO in order to apply for the Medicare Shared Savings Program (MSSP). The physicians and hospital system are each equal owners of the ACO. The clinically integrated WEHC IPA, representing 430 physicians in 100 groups, had received P4P reimbursement for many years. All commercial payers saw value in rolling their contracts into the ACO along with the MSSP. Accordingly, the legacy physician incentive programs were also carried over into the ACO.

David Cook, chief administrative officer, notes that the MSSP requirement of a separate entity adds complication because any MSSP check goes to the ACO. The ACO is then responsible for distributing incentives to physician groups, who then distribute to individual physicians. The group compensation formula should support the incentives of the whole system and the goal of shared savings.

Each of the 100 groups in the IPA determines their own compensation models. Cook encourages the groups to align their physician compensation plans with the ACO goals and incentives. For example, when one group contemplated paying the quality bonus based on production, he talked with them about maintaining alignment with the quality and outcomes strategies of the ACO, which they ultimately did. This group retained 30 percent of the incentive payment to cover infrastructure support for chronic disease management and paid 70 percent to the physicians as calculated by the ACO.

The ACO's physician incentive program contains two pools determined each year by the ACO board depending on the amount of funds received from payers. The two pools are:

1. Physician profile pool; and

2. Chronic care pool.

The profile pool is based on the physician scorecard developed by the ACO. The physicians are ranked according to a 100-point score system and paid a flat dollar amount when certain thresholds are reached. Cook said 15–20 percent of physicians don't achieve thresholds and don't receive any incentive dollars, while 10–20 percent receive the highest amount for top scores in the profile.

The Physician Performance Profile is reviewed once a year to ensure that it aligns with the clinical integration plan approved annually by the ACO board. In 2012, the profile and incentive program included five domains; a sixth was added in 2013. The 2013 domains are:

1. Patient quality, based on specialty-specific measures.

2. Efficiency or cost measures, including measures that are components in standard protocols and shared savings under Medicare Advantage participation. Examples include generic drug utilization, rates of unnecessary imaging and testing, and complying with a low-back-pain algorithm to reduce surgical procedures.

3. Patient satisfaction.

4. Patient safety. This was added relatively recently and emphasizes inpatient factors including inpatient falls and hospital-acquired infections. There are not as many physician office safety measures at this time.

5. Patient access, measuring the number of patients seen without insurance or on Medicaid.

6. Community benefit. This was added in 2013 to promote physician volunteer efforts in the community like volunteering in a free community clinic.

Some measures or metrics in each domain apply to every physician, while others are specialty specific or dependent on payer contracts. Extra credit points are typically added each year for a particular issue selected by organization leadership. Interestingly, this tends to generate more discussion than other factors.

Another factor that the Physician Performance Profile reviews is citizenship or accountable care engagement. This component rates physician participation in various work groups and other ACO meetings. Participation is important to the ACO because of emphasis on clinical integration and the need to reach agreement on medical protocols.

The chronic care pool is determined by the number of successful patients that physicians have in their panels. Successful patients are those with chronic diseases or other health issues that the physician has helped stabilize or improve. The higher the number of chronic care patients in a physician's panel, the greater the opportunity to receive more reward.

The following is an example of "successful patient" determination: Physician A has 100 diabetics, while Physician B has 50. Physician B successfully manages blood pressure on 45 of the patients but Physician A only achieves successful management with 30. Physician B receives more income since she has a higher number of patients with a controlled blood pressure.

The chronic care pool is distributed in this manner because payers look at the results for the total patient panel in order to encourage improvement of a large percentage of chronic care patients. Therefore, physicians with a large number of chronic care patients receive more in incentive payments from the payer. Currently, there are two physicians in the IPA who are doing extremely well in managing more than 100 diabetics in their patient panels.

This incentive calculation is still controversial because physicians with a high percentage of success but fewer patients complain that their success rate isn't rewarded. Cook believes this method provides the incentive to accept more chronic care patients and ensure physicians are doing the right thing for more people. The organization can't accept that it's okay for some patients to be managed better than others. The more patients there are with better outcomes, the more funds that will be available for rewarding physicians.

The organization is still moving toward team-based care, especially with Medicare patients. They are hiring health coaches to support Johns Hopkins' "guided care" model as an alternative to PCMH rather than dealing with NCQA (National Committee for Quality Assurance) certification. The ACO will be hiring and paying for the additional staff. The increase in staff costs may initially impact the dollars available to physicians, but the expectation is that new staff will improve scores and payer rating, resulting in more dollars to fund physician compensation in the future.

Things to think about: David Cook realizes that FFS continues as the major factor, so incentives to maintain productivity are needed while including quality as a component. Healthcare organizations will need more complex formulas in the future to address quality factors while maintaining productivity. Cook describes the ProHealth solution for receiving value-based reimbursement: "We built the aqueduct which doesn't have a lot flowing through it right now but is capable of handling double or triple that flow." He advises:

> Organizations need to set up the system now and be comfortable with the increase in P4P in the future. ACOs can count on earning more dollars now through payer incentives but some will evolve to have downside consequences. In a few more years, penalties could be a factor. If the ACO suffers penalties in the future, where does the money come from? Physician compensation may have to add downside risk in future. Physician compensation might be withheld until thresholds are achieved leaving more uncertainty for physicians.

Additional Integrated System Models

Advocate Health System[18]

Advocate Health System, a 12-hospital system based in Chicago with 3,800 employed physicians, developed one set of metrics to rate and reward its employed and affiliated physicians. This enables the system to negotiate with payers based on its criteria rather than how the various insurers had chosen to judge its performance. The compensation incentive program is described as follows:

> *Starting with 36 measures in 2004, Advocate rewarded its affiliated and employed physicians for performance and adherence to the standards via a clinical integration incentive fund to which most of its insurers contribute. Each physician receives compensation related to both his or her own performance as well as the overall performance of other members of the physician–hospital organization. Today, Advocate has roughly 150 measures in place; its incentive payouts to physicians grew from $12.4 million in 2005 to $50 million in 2010.*

Mark Shields, MD, senior medical director for Advocate Physician Partners, the system's care management venture with its employed physicians, says, "Advocate was able to convince its insurers that the use of a standard set of measures would engage and motivate physicians and other clinicians."

Mount Auburn Hospital[19]

Mount Auburn Hospital, based in Cambridge, Mass., is a smaller organization, with around 160 physicians, than many described here but still shares the belief that physician incentives work. According to Jeanette Clough, president and CEO, "Everyone is on incentives because the physician should not be divorced from the realities of running a practice."

Compensation for PCPs is based on annual goals of patient visits and net revenue to reflect the importance to balance productivity incentive while maintaining the focus on patient care. If productivity goals are not achieved, then only 10 percent of the base salary is at risk, which rarely occurs. Revenues above the goal are split 50-50 between physician and hospital. Adjustments are made depending on the socioeconomic status of the neighborhood where physicians serve. Bonuses for quality and efficiency are funded from payers' incentives after the money has passed through hospital accounts. Clough stated that there are special incentive programs for OB/GYN and emergency physicians because of differences in their specialties.

Large Multispecialty Practices[20]

Although the following case studies described by Alice G. Gosfield, Esq., a healthcare lawyer, are a few years old, they give excellent examples of incentive plans in large group practices.

PriMed, a physician multispecialty group with more than 60 physicians in Dayton, Ohio, began incentive compensation based on physician compliance with hypertension treatment standards. The program was introduced with an education component to prepare the physicians, and there was no withhold or incentive payment the first year. The initial withhold of 3 percent of gross revenues to fund the incentive pool grew to 5 percent. The process was introduced incrementally, one measure at a time, and added diabetes treatment protocol adherence over time. At the time of the interview, they were shifting toward a model with 95 percent compensation based on productivity and 5 percent on quality. A total of about $10,000 per physician was at risk depending on quality and/or citizenship factors.

HealthCare Partners Medical Group is a combination of medical practices and IPAs with more than 400 physicians practicing in 40 offices in Southern California. Compensation metrics for PCPs are directly linked to P4P incentives from payers. In 2006–2007, these measures included breast and cervical cancer screening, HbA1c control, and LDL control. Total compensation determination also factors in productivity measures, patient satisfaction, and managed care panel size (weighted by gender, age, and continuity).

The Camino Medical Group in northern California is a 180-physician multispecialty group that is part of the Sutter Health network. They award the top half of their physicians a discretionary bonus of generally $1,000 to $3,000 per year, based on a single blended score of internally collected peer review data and patient satisfaction scores. The decision of final distribution is based on physician performance scores, comparative performance with the group's physicians, and the discretion of the medical director.

Duluth Clinic in Minnesota, a 425-physician group, uses compensation pool distribution (not bonuses) controlled at the section level. Each section decides the compensation calculation based on factors such as service within the section, and clinical and operational excellence goals. The group emphasizes team metrics since leadership and culture are seen as the primary factors in organizational success, supported by compensation methodology. As an example for hospitalists, 9 percent of each physician's salary depends on a group incentive pool with two goals: (1) achieve the cardiology measures at more than 60 percent accuracy; and (2) reduce the average length of stay for their top ten disease-related groups by 0.2 days or more.

Partners HealthCare in Boston (Mass.), a large, integrated system, participates in value-based performance contracts with its major payers. The payers withhold a portion of reimbursement until the system as a whole meets its targets. Targets include HEDIS scores, use of computerized physician order entry and electronic health records, and managing costs. Partners in Boston measures and reports physicians' progress relative to the P4P targets. Specialty-specific goals are emphasized, including "lowering high-cost imaging for the radiologists, managing drug use more effectively for dermatologists, and meeting HEDIS standards for diabetic care for primary physicians and endocrinologists."

The compensation formula for Health Partners in Minneapolis, Minn., bases 90 percent of compensation on productivity and 10 percent on patient satisfaction, quality, and participation (citizenship). The quality metrics have moved toward outcome-based measures, including the goals of 20 percent of patients with diabetes having HbA1c and LDL results below specific measures, or percentage of patients with blood pressure below 130. The incentive pools are funded by setting aside increases in the market compensation rates per wRVU each year rather than withholding a part of total reimbursement. Leaders credit a part of their success to demonstrating to physicians the importance of quality as an organizational goal.

End Notes

1. Donna Knapp, MA, FACMPE, personal conversation with authors, April 10, 2013.
2. Jennifer L. Souders, FACMPE, "Establishing a Physician Compensation Plan," ACMPE Fellow Paper (October 2011), http://www.mgma.com/workarea/mgma_downloadasset.aspx?id=1368495.
3. William R. Greenfield, MD, "In Search of an Effective Physician Compensation Formula," *Family Practice Management*, 5, no.9 (1998): 50–57.
4. Debbie A. Kiehl, "Redesign of the Employed Physicians Compensation Model," ACMPE Fellowship Paper (October 2011).
5. Alice G Gosfield, Esq., "Compensating Physicians for Quality and Value: A Changing Landscape," *Group Practice Journal*, 60, no.8 (2011): 16–26.
6. Robert L. Bratton, MD, "Salaried vs. Productivity-Based Physician Compensation: Advantages and Pitfalls," *Group Practice Journal*, 59, no.8 (2010): 38–48.
7. David Taylor, vice president, Regional Services (Integrated Physicians Group), CoxHealth, personal conversation with author February 11, 2013.
8. Karen Minich-Pourshadi, "Group Practice Innovators: Investing in Success," *HealthLeaders Media* (September 13, 2011), https://www.healthleadersmedia.com/page-5/MAG-270671/Group-Practice-Innovators-Investing-in-Success (accessed April 25, 2013).
9. Craig E. Samitt, MD, "Rewarding Better Care at Lower Cost: Re-Designing MD Compensation in the World of Accountable Care" (presentation at Health Industry Forum, October 22, 2012), http://healthforum.brandeis.edu/meetings/materials/2012-22-oct-CAPP1/2SamittHIF102212.pdf.pdf (accessed April 25, 2013).
10. Jim Molpus, "How Dean Clinic Redesigned Primary Care," *HealthLeaders Media* (April 22, 2013), http://www.healthleadersmedia.com/page-1/COM-291352/How-Dean-Clinic-Redesigned-Primary-Care (accessed April 25, 2013).

11. Steven Pierdon and Brenda Eckrote, "Changing Compensation Plans Moving Beyond Last Year's, This Year's and Next Year's," *Physician Executive*, 30, no.1 (2004): 26–29.

12. Steven Pierdon and Brenda Eckrote, "Transforming Care Delivery: Patient-Centric, Value-Driven Innovation," *Group Practice Journal*, 61, no.4, (2012): 19–20, 26–31.

13. T.D. Lee, "How Geisinger Structures Its Physicians' Compensation to Support Improvements in Quality, Efficiency, and Volume," *Health Affairs*, 31, no.9 (2012): 2068–2073.

14. Christine A. Schon, vice president, Community Group Practices, Dartmouth-Hitchcock, personal communication with author, March 18, 2013.

15. Willie Rainey Jr. and Chrissy van Erkelens, "Genuine Quality and Service Incentives in a Physician P4P Program," *Group Practice Journal*, 59, no.8 (2010): 21–27.

16. Stephen Nuckolls, CEO, Coastal Carolina Health Care, P.A., conversation with author, March 6, 2013.

17. David Cook, chief administrative officer, ProHealth Solutions, Wisconsin, personal conversation with author, March 6, 2013.

18. H. Haydn Bush, "A Health System Convinces Insurers to Play by Its Quality Rules," *H&HN: Hospitals & Health Networks*, 85, no.8 (2011): 13.

19. Lola Butcher, "Financial Incentives for employed Physicians: Do They Work?" *PEJ*, July 36, no.4 (2010): 18–21.

20. Alice G. Gosfield, "Chapter 1: Physician Compensation for Quality: Behind the Group's Green Door," *Health Law Handbook,* Sec. 1.6 (2008 edition), 3–44, http://www.gosfield.com/PDF/Published.Chapter1.pdf (accessed February 8, 2013).

Additional Resources

MGMA-ACMPE Resources (www.mgma.com)	
Resource	**Website Location**
Physician compensation resources, articles, webinars, etc.	Listed under Practice Resources
Physician Compensation and Production Survey, Cost Survey, and other surveys and benchmark reports	Industry Data
Procedural Profile Module	Industry Data
Stark law, Medicare regulations, and reimbursement, etc.	Government Affairs
Books, webinars, other resources	MGMA-ACMPE Store
Online discussion forums	Membership, Member Community
Non-MGMA-ACMPE articles, FAQs, research assistance	Knowledge Center, listed under Additional Resources
MGMA Health Care Consulting Group	Consulting

Government Resources

Resource	Website
Centers for Medicare & Medicaid Services (CMS)	www.cms.gov
Center for Medicare & Medicaid Innovation (CMMI)	http://innovation.cms.gov
CMS Physician Quality Reporting System (PQRS)	www.cms.gov/Medicare/Quality-Initiatives-Patient-Assessment-Instruments/PQRS/index.html
CMS, Quality Improvement Organizations information	www.cms.gov/QualityImprovementOrgs
CMS electronic health record (EHR) Incentive Programs (Meaningful Use)	www.cms.gov/EHRIncentivePrograms
Agency for Healthcare Research and Quality (AHRQ)— One AHRQ initiative is the Comparative Effectiveness Research (CER), which looks at the difference in costs and outcomes of various treatment options for the same conditions.	www.ahrq.gov
National Quality Measures Clearinghouse	www.qualitymeasures.ahrq.gov
National Guidelines Clearinghouse	www.guideline.gov
AHRQ's Consumer Assessment of Healthcare Providers and Systems (CG-CAHPS) Clinician & Group Surveys	www.cahps.ahrq.gov/clinician_group

Patient-Centered Medical Home

Resource	Website
Bridges to Excellence, a project led by a coalition of major U.S. businesses; includes Medical Home Recognition Project	www.bridgestoexcellence.org
HealthTeamWorks promotes the adoption of evidence-based clinical guidelines in practice; assists with the implementation and use of technology, such as electronic health records and patient registries; and facilitates the transition from traditional healthcare to the patient-centered medical home (PCMH).	www.healthteamworks.org
National Committee for Quality Assurance (NCQA) certifies medical groups under the Physician Organization certification program and the Physician Practice Connections–Patient-Centered Medical Home.	www.ncqa.org
TransforMED, a subsidiary of the American Academy of Family Physicians, "acts as a leader and a catalyst to generate positive transformations in family medicine and primary care." They also offer a series of PCMH workbooks for medical practices.	www.transformed.com

Quality Measures and Guidelines

Resource	Website
Accreditation Association for Ambulatory Health Care (AAAHC) develops "standards to advance and promote patient safety, quality care, and value for ambulatory healthcare through peer-based accreditation processes, education, and research." The AAAHC Institute for Quality Improvement is involved in clinical performance measurement tools designed specifically for the ambulatory care environment. AAAHC also offers medical home certification.	www.aaahc.org
Ambulatory Quality Alliance (AQA) is a joint effort of the American Academy of Family Physicians (AAFP), the American College of Physicians (ACP), America's Health Insurance Plans (AHIP), and the Agency for Healthcare Research and Quality (AHRQ).	www.ambulatoryqualityalliance.org
America's Health Insurance Plans (AHIP) provides healthcare quality resources.	www.ahip.org/Issues/Health-Care -Quality.aspx
American Medical Association–Physician Consortium for Performance Improvement (AMA-PCPI) was developed to enhance the "quality of care and patient safety by taking the lead in the development, testing, and maintenance of evidence-based clinical performance measures and measurement resources for physicians." It is comprised of medical specialty societies, state medical societies, the American Board of Medical Specialties, professional organizations, and federal agencies. It was instrumental in developing many quality measurements used by the CMS's PQRS.	http://www.ama-assn.org/go/pcpi
Health Care Incentives Improvement Institute (HCI3)	www.hci3.org
Prometheus Payment	http://www.hci3.org/what_is_prometheus
Institute for Healthcare Improvement works with The Joint Commission on Accreditation of Healthcare Organizations and other quality organizations to standardize pay-for-performance measures and evidence-based practices.	www.ihi.org
National Association for Healthcare Quality is dedicated to the advancement of the profession of healthcare quality and patient safety and the individual professionals working in the field.	www.nahq.org

Table continued next page

Quality Measures and Guidelines (continued)

Resource	Website
National Center for Quality Assurance (NCQA) places emphasis on certifying managed care organizations. It developed the Healthcare Effectiveness Data and Information Set (HEDIS), standardized measures to simplify comparing healthcare performance of managed care plans. NCQA developed many of the clinical quality measures used in the CMS PQRS program.	www.ncqa.org
National Quality Forum (NQF) is also working to standardize healthcare quality measures and ensure consistent evidence-based practices and comparable data. Many of their endorsed healthcare performance measures were adopted by CMS.	www.qualityforum.org
URAC accredits health plans, preferred provider organizations, and other healthcare organizations. It is involved with the "development of quantitative measures for accreditation programs and the analysis and reporting of measure results." URAC also offers a Patient Centered Health Care (Medical) Home (PCHCH) Program.	www.urac.org

Understanding RVUs and the RBRVS System

The resource-based relative value scale (RBRVS) is a system used by the Centers for Medicare & Medicaid Services (CMS) to determine reimbursement rates or fees for physician services under Medicare. The RBRVS includes an assigned relative value unit (RVU) value for each Current Procedural Terminology® (CPT®)[*] code (developed by the American Medical Association). The RBRVS system was developed by Dr. William C. Hsiao of the Harvard School of Public Health and approved for use in support of Medicare physician payments by the Omnibus Budget Reconciliation Act of 1989.

The RBRVS system does not include any consideration for actual practice costs or severity of illness, quality of care, demand for services, or healthcare outcomes. It is based on the perceived value of each service relative to other physician services.

The three RVU components used to calculate the total RVU are as follows:

1. Work RVUs (wRVUs) measure the time and effort of the provider in the delivery of a service or procedure. This includes preparation time, waiting time, presurgery activities, time during interaction between the provider and the patient (the surgery or appointment time), and post-service time including follow-up care. The wRVU factors in the provider's mental effort, technical skill, physical effort, and stress involved in delivering the service. The higher the complexity and time, then the greater the wRVU value.

2. Practice expense RVU (peRVU) incorporates the average expected direct and indirect costs of the medical practice required to complete the procedure or service.

3. Malpractice expense RVU (meRVU) factors in the relative risk to the provider and the relative cost of training related to the specialty that performs the specific service. It is not actually based on the cost of malpractice insurance.

---

[*] CPT © 2014 American Medical Association. All rights reserved.

The three components are adjusted by the Geographic Adjustment Factor (GAF) to compensate for differences among geographic regions within the United States. The GAF in turn is separated into three components called Geographic Practice Cost Indices or GPCIs. Each RVU component has its own GPCI and is used to calculate the total RVU:

Geographically Adjusted Total RVU = [(Work RVU × Work GPCI)wGPCI]
+ (Practice Expense RVU × Practice Expense GPCI [peGPCI])
+ (Malpractice Expense RVU × Malpractice Expense GPCI [meGPCI])]

The final Medicare Physician Fee Schedule (MPFS) is determined by multiplying the geographically adjusted RVUs by the Medicare conversion factor (CF).

$$\text{Fee} = \text{RVU}_{TOT} \times \text{Medicare CF}[1]$$

The following calculation is an example using procedure code 99213 for parts of Florida:

[(wRVU× wGPCI) + (peRVU × peGPCI) + (meRVU × meGPCI)] =
0.097 × 1.00 + 1.03 × 0.968 + 0.07 × 0.553 =
0.097 + 0.997 + 0.0387 = 1.133 Geographically Adjusted Total RVUs

The Medicare Physician Fee Schedule MPFS CF for 2013 is $34.0230: 1.133 × $34.0230 = $38.54.[2] This is the amount that Medicare will reimburse for 99213 in areas of Florida.

To sum up the calculation, the fee for a CPT code is based on total RVUs (physician work, practice expense, and malpractice expense RVUs) multiplied by the geographic adjustment and the CF, which is determined each year. Total reimbursement from Medicare is based on the groups' total fees for a patient's service. Many payers use the MPFS adjusted to a percentage of Medicare's fees (i.e., reimburse at 115 percent of Medicare) or they use a proprietary fee schedule.

The Medicare CF for each year is announced toward the end of the previous year based on the sustainable growth rate (SGR) formula. Enacted by the Balanced Budget Act of 1997, it was intended to ensure that the yearly increase in the expense per Medicare beneficiary does not exceed the growth in gross domestic product. If the expenditures for the previous year exceeded the target expenditures, then the conversion factor will decrease payments for the next year. However, the SGR is considered to be a flawed method and requires votes every year to avoid the deep cuts in Medicare payments to physicians required by the formula. The Medicare Payment Advisory Commission and healthcare stakeholders, including MGMA, have proposed various alternatives for fixing the system, but Congress hasn't approved any proposals.

The RVU values for each CPT code are determined by the Relative Value Update Committee, an American Medical Association–affiliated private committee that tends to be specialty biased. Meetings are closed, so there is uncertainty on determination of values and future influences and changes. For this reason, groups may want to consider modifying the RVU values in the physician compensation formula. For example, multispecialty practices can increase the values for certain primary care office visits and services to recognize the value that primary care physicians play in managing patient care and chronic disease management goals. As an example, one radiology practice increased the value of basic X-ray readings so its physicians would be encouraged for providing the much needed, basic services.

Private/Commercial Payers Fee Schedules

Private payers use the CMS RBRVS system or other fee schedules for determining their reimbursement rates for physician and other outpatient services. These systems will include CPT codes for services not included in the RBRVS since Medicare only serves a population of 65 years of age and older. Relative value scales that are still used by some commercial payers include California RVUs and Florida RVUs. *Relative Values for Physicians* (RVP), published by Optum (previously known as Ingenix), is an RVU scale that was developed for insurers and for physicians to develop their own fee schedules.

End Notes

1. Frank Cohen, MBB, MPA: *RVUs: Applications for Medical Practice Success*, 3rd ed. (Englewood, CO: Medical Group Management Association, 2013).
2. Ibid.

Compensation per Work RVU Ratio Selection[1]

As mentioned in chapter 3, the dollar figure representing compensation per work relative value unit (wRVU) ratios is often used in compensation formulas based on wRVUs. A selected ratio is multiplied by the number of wRVUs for the pay period to determine physicians' compensation. Surveys, like the MGMA Physician Compensation and Production Survey, are frequently used to determine a fair ratio to calculate compensation.

In these surveys, figures are typically presented in tables showing the median and various percentiles. The tendency in using benchmarking data is to select higher percentiles (75th or 90th percentiles) in compensation and production figures to provide goals and incentives for physicians to achieve high performance. For example, practices who want to compensate physicians at the 75th percentile, especially if their production is at the 75th percentile, will look at compensation per wRVU at the 75th percentile. Using the data from the example in Exhibit C.1, a practice may use $81.01 for the compensation per wRVU ratio. With compensation per wRVU ratios, this practice will backfire because the higher percentiles actually reflect highly compensated physicians relative to the number of RVUs. These physicians may be on guaranteed salaries or other compensation that is not based on the number of RVUs.

EXHIBIT C.1 ■ Sample Compensation to Work RVU Analysis

	10th Percentile	25th Percentile	Median	75th Percentile	90th Percentile
Reported compensation	$237,971	$345,647	$455,762	$616,400	$837,834
Reported wRVU	4,128	6,071	7,966	10,924	13,235
Reported compensation per wRVU	$38.60	$47.97	$59.00	$81.01	$104.95

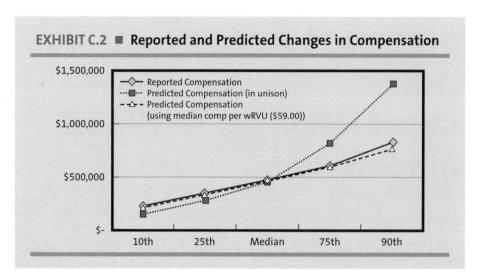

EXHIBIT C.2 ■ **Reported and Predicted Changes in Compensation**

As Exhibit C.2 shows, if compensation was determined by multiplying physicians' reported wRVUs by the compensation per wRVU value for the reported percentile, then compensation would follow the predicted compensation line shown in Exhibit C.1. As shown, the compensation at the 10th and 25th percentile is lower than reported compensation, and the compensation at the 90th percentile would actually be $500,000 higher than the median compensation reported in the MGMA report. However, if reported wRVUs are multiplied by the median compensation per wRVU ratio, the calculated compensation closely mirrors the actual reported compensation.

Plotting actual compensation per wRVU compared with compensation, as shown in Exhibit C.3, shows a reverse J-shaped curve. As production and compensation rise, this graph demonstrates how the compensation per wRVU ratio decreases. The highest percentiles of compensation per wRVU actually reflect the lowest producers since they have a relatively high compensation compared to the actual wRVUs they generate.

Another thing to keep in mind when using MGMA compensation survey data is the great variety of methods used in determining compensation among respondents to the survey. Many practices and health systems that provide survey data use methods other than productivity-based compensation plans, thereby affecting the nature of the compensation and wRVU results.

Practice executives are advised to use the median compensation per wRVU value from the survey report tables as a base for calculating compensation. When physicians increase their productivity and number of wRVUs, their compensation will increase even if the compensation per wRVU remains the same as seen in Exhibit C.2. Several other options (discussed further in chapter 3) can be used to provide incentives for higher wRVU production:

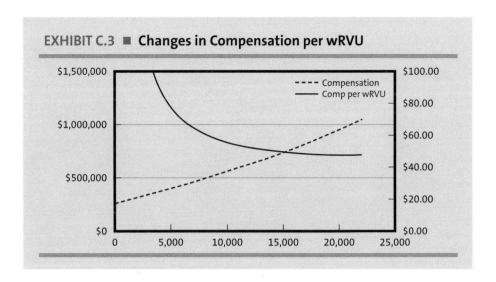

EXHIBIT C.3 ■ **Changes in Compensation per wRVU**

1. Straight line increase in compensation per wRVU values as compensation increases;

2. Base salary plus bonus based on wRVUs; and

3. Tiered plans with compensation per wRVU value increasing as preset points of physician productivity levels.

End Note

1. Todd B. Evenson, MBA, "The Relationship of Compensation to Production," MGMA presentation, June 28, 2012, shared with author, January 2013.

Bibliography

Agency for Health Care Policy and Research. "Theory and Reality of Value-Based Purchasing: Lessons from the Pioneers," AHCPR Publication No. 98-0004, Rockville, MD: Agency for Health Care Policy and Research, November 1997, http://www.ahrq.gov/qual/meyerrpt.htm (accessed February 25, 2013).

Baker, Marshall. "Physician Compensation – Addressing the Gray Areas." MGMA webinar, November 10, 2011.

Berry, Emily. "Private Shared-Savings Deal Puts Half of Future Raises at Hospital System at Risk." *amednews*, July 31, 2012, http://www.ama-assn.org/amed news/2012/07/30/bisd0731.htm (accessed February 14, 2013).

Berry, Emily. "What's Behind WellPoint's Pay Raise for Primary Care Doctors?" *amednews*, February 13, 2012, http://www.ama-assn.org/amednews/2012/02/13/ bisb0213.htm (accessed February 15, 2013).

Berwick, Donald M., Thomas W. Nolan, and John Whittington. "The Triple Aim: Care, Health, and Cost," IHI Innovation Series White Paper. Cambridge, Mass: Institute for Healthcare Improvement (2012), http://content.healthaffairs.org/ content/27/3/759.long (accessed February 28, 2013).

Bloom Jr., Frederick J., MD, MMM. "Transforming Care Delivery: Patient-Centric, Value-Driven Innovation." *Group Practice Journal*, 61, no.4 (2012): 19–20, 26–31.

Bohlmann, Robert C., FACMPE. "Is Your Integration a Marriage of Equals?" *MGMA Directions*, Spring 2012, pp. 4–5, http://www.mgma.com/WorkArea/mgma_down loadasset.aspx?id=1370965 (accessed March 12, 2013).

Bokur, Debra. "Can Global Payment Improve on Fee for Service and Capitation and Lower Healthcare Costs?" *MGMA Connexion* supplement, "How to Get Paid," May/June 2012, http://www.mgma.com/workarea/mgma_downloadasset.aspx ?id=1370833 (accessed March 2, 2013).

Bratton, Robert L., MD. "Salaried vs. Productivity-Based Physician Compensation: Advantages and Pitfalls." *Group Practice Journal*, 59, no.8 (2010): 38–43.

Bush, H. Haydn. "A Health System Convinces Insurers to Play by Its Quality Rules." *H&HN: Hospitals & Health Networks*, 85, no.8 (2011): 13.

Butcher, Lola. "Financial Incentives for Employed Physicians: Do They Work?" *PEJ*, 36, no.4 (2012): 18–21.

Chamblee, Justin, CPA. "Future Concepts in Physician Compensation." Presentation, MGMA Financial Management and Payer Contracting Conference, Phoenix, AZ, February 25–26, 2013.

Chamblee, Justin, CPA. "Physician Compensation: Design a Plan That Responds to Integration and Alignment." MGMA Financial Management and Payer Contracting Conference, Phoenix, AZ, February 24–26, 2013.

Cohen, Frank, MPA. *RVUs: Applications for Medical Practice Success*, 3rd Edition. Englewood, CO: Medical Group Management Association, 2013.

Cohen, Frank, MPA. "Using Work RVUs to Compensate Docs: A Bomb-Proof Methodology." Presentation, MGMA Financial Management and Payer Contracting Conference, Phoenix, AZ, February 24–26, 2013.

Davis, Shawana Lynn, FACMPE. "Using Benchmark Data to Evaluate Overall Practice Position." ACMPE Fellowship Paper, 2011, http://www.mgma.com/workarea/downloadasset.aspx?id=1368531 (accessed February 12, 2013).

Driscoll, M. "Physician Acquisition: What to Avoid After the Deal Is Complete." *hfm (Healthcare Financial Management)*, 66, no.4 (2012): 90–94.

Elliott, Victoria Stagg. "3 Steps to Quality Pay for Physicians." *amednews*, July 23, 2012, http://www.ama-assn.org/amednews/2012/07/23/bisa0723.htm (accessed February 14, 2013).

Elliott, Victoria Stagg. "Hospitals Behind Physician Recruiting for Not-So-Solo Practices." *amednews*, posted July 23, 2012, http://www.ama-assn.org/amednews/2012/07/23/bil20723.htm (accessed February 14, 2013).

Elliott, Victoria Stagg. "Physician Employment: Build a Contract That Suits You." *amednews*, January 14, 2013, http://www.ama-assn.org/amednews/2013/01/14/bisa0114.htm (accessed February 14, 2013).

Emerman, Charles L., MD, Jonathan Siff, MD, and Alfred F. Connors Jr., MD. "Hospital Reaps Rewards from RVU Incentive-Based Program." *MGMA Connexion*, November/December 2010, https://www.mgma.com/workarea/mgma_downloadasset.aspx?id=40204 (accessed February 26, 2013).

Enos, Nancy M. "RVUs Are Your Biggest Chips in Physician-Employment Bargaining." *MGMA e-Source*, March 13, 2012, http://mgma.com/article.aspx?id=1370192 (accessed February 12, 2013).

Evenson, Todd B. "New Trends in Physician Compensation Planning." MGMA webinar, April 18, 2013.

Fabrizio, Nick A., PhD, FACMPE, with Robert C. Bohlmann, FACMPE. *Integrated Delivery Systems: Ensuring Successful Physician-Hospital Partnerships.* Englewood, CO: Medical Group Management Association, 2010.

Fiegl, Charles. "Medicare Pay: Insurers Preview a Post-SGR World." *amednews,* February 4, 2013, http://www.ama-assn.org/amednews/2013/02/04/gvsa0204 .htm (accessed February 14, 2013).

Fowler, Todd M., FACMPE. "From Recruiting to Provider Relations – A Mission-Critical Transformation." ACMPE Fellowship Paper, October 2011.

Franco, Miranda. "Evaluating Medicare ACOs and Bundled Payment Initiatives." *MGMA Connexion,* January 2013, pp. 35–36.

Gans, David N., MSHA, FACMPE. "Data Mine: Keeping Up with Inflation." *MGMA Connexion,* January 2011, http://www.mgma.com/workarea/mgma_download asset.aspx?id=40536 (accessed February 12, 2013).

Gans, David N., MSHA, FACMPE. "Data Mine: What Drives Physician Salaries?" *MGMA Connexion,* October 2012, https://mgma.com/workarea/mgma_download asset.aspx?id=1372057 (accessed February 15, 2013).

Gans, David N., MSHA, FACMPE. "Data Mine: Why Hospital-Owned Medical Groups Lose Money." *MGMA Connexion,* April 2012, http://mgma.com/workarea/ mgma_downloadasset.aspx?id=1370391 (accessed February 21, 2013).

Gans, David N., MSHA, FACMPE. "Preparing for Value-Based Payment." Presentation, MGMA Financial Management and Payer Contracting Conference, Phoenix, AZ, February 25–26, 2013.

Gans, David N., MSHA, FACMPE. "What You Reward, You Get – And Lots of It." *MGMA Connexion,* 10, no.2 (2010): 17–18.

Gans, David N., MSHA, FACMPE. "With Increasing Costs, How Do Practices Maintain Their Bottom Line?" *MGMA Connexion,* January 2013, http://www .mgma.com/workarea/mgma_downloadasset.aspx?id=1373084 (accessed February 20, 2013).

Gans, David N., MSHA, FACMPE. "You Don't Know What You Don't Know: Information Needs for Future Payment Systems." Presentation, MGMA Financial Management and Payer Contracting Conference, Phoenix, AZ, February 25–26, 2013.

Gosfield, Alice G. "Chapter 1: Physician Compensation for Quality: Behind the Group's Green Door." *Health Law Handbook,* Sec. 1.6, 2008 edition, pp. 3–44. http://www.gosfield.com/PDF/Published.Chapter1.pdf (accessed February 8, 2013).

Gosfield, Alice G., Esq. "Compensating Physicians for Quality and Value: A Changing Landscape." *Group Practice Journal,* 60, no.8 (2011): 16–26.

Greenfield, William R., MD. "In Search of an Effective Physician Compensation Formula." *Family Practice Management,* 5, no.9 (1998): 50–57.

Guglielmo, Wayne J. "This Doctor Made P4P Work – You Can Too." *Medical Economics*, 85, no.14 (2008): 34-6, 42-4.

Helmchen, Lorens A., and Anthony T. Lo Sasso. "How Sensitive Is Physician Performance to Alternative Compensation Schedules? Evidence from a Large Network of Primary Care Clinics." *Health Economics*, 19 (2010): 1300–1317.

Heymans, Mary. "Physician Leadership Incentive Compensation Plans." *Becker's Hospital Review*, June 14, 2011, http://www.beckershospitalreview.com/compensation-issues/physician-leadership-incentive-compensation-plans.html (accessed April 22, 2013).

Hill, Alan. "Show Me the Money: Developing the Right Compensation Structure for Your Practice." *MGMA Connexion*, August 2010, https://mgma.com/workarea/mgma_downloadasset.aspx?id=34424 (accessed February 10, 2013).

Huang, Elbert S., and Kenneth Finegold. "Seven Million Americans Live in Areas Where Demand for Primary Care May Exceed Supply by More Than 10 Percent." *Health Affairs*, 32 (2013): 614–621.

James, Marcia. "Successful Partnerships in Practice: A Payer Perspective." *MGMA Connexion*, 13, no.4 (2013): 38–40.

Johnson, Bruce A., JD, MPA, and Deborah Walker Keegan. *Physician Compensation Plans: State of the Art Strategies*. Englewood, CO: Medical Group Management Association, 2006, p. 235.

Kasher, Mick, and David Fein. "Benchmarking Physician Compensation and Production: Data Dive Compensation Module." MGMA webinar, January 28, 2009, https://mgmameetings.webex.com/mgmameetings/lsr.php?AT=pb&SP=EC&rID=5944532&rKey=f5ea63b538369984 (accessed January 22, 2013).

Kiehl, Debbie A. "Redesign of the Employed Physicians Compensation Model." ACMPE Fellowship Paper, October 2011.

Laugesen, M.J., and S.A. Glied. "Higher Fees Paid to US Physicians Drive Higher Spending for Physician Services Compared to Other Countries." *Health Affairs* 30 (2011): 1647–1656.

Lee, T.D. "How Geisinger Structures Its Physicians' Compensation to Support Improvements in Quality, Efficiency, and Volume." *Health Affairs*, 31, no.9 (2012): 2068–2073.

Leonard, Devin. "Medicare and Medicaid Must Be Cut. Period." *Business Week*, November 8, 2012, http://www.businessweek.com/articles/2012-11-08/medicare-and-medicaid-must-be-cut-dot-period (accessed February 22, 2013).

Levine, J.K. "Compensation Models and Issues for a Multispecialty Group Practice." *Journal of Ambulatory Care Management*, 19(1996): 50–59.

Lowes, Robert. "1 in 4 Physicians Employed by Large Groups Are Part-Time." *Medscape Medical News*, March 21, 2012, http://www.cejkasearch.com/wp-content/uploads/Medscape_03.21_-1-in-4-Physicians-Are-Part-Time.pdf (accessed March 12, 2013).

"Meaningful Use EHR Incentive Payments Near $13 Billion," *MGMA Washington Connexion*, April 17, 2013.

Mechanic, Robert, and Darren E. Zinner. "Many Large Medical Groups Will Need to Acquire New Skills and Tools to Be Ready for Payment Reform." *Health Affairs*, 31, no.9 (2012): 1984–1992.

Mechanic, Robert, Palmira Santos, Bruce Landon, and Michael Chernew. "Medical Group Responses to Global Payment: Early Lessons from the 'Alternative Quality Contract' in Massachusetts." *Health Affairs*, 30, no.9 (2011): 1734–1742.

Medical Group Management Association. "FAQs: Data Calculations and Glossary." MGMA Physician Compensation and Production Survey definitions. http://www.mgma.com/pm/default.aspx?id=9252 (accessed March 10, 2013).

Medical Group Management Association. *MGMA Patient-Centered Care: 2012 Status and Prospects Report*. Englewood, CO: MGMA-ACMPE, 2012.

Medical Group Management Association, "State of Medical Practice – Integrated Delivery Systems." *MGMA Connexion*, January 2010, www.mgma.com/workarea/downloadasset.aspx?id=32156 (accessed April 27, 2013).

Medical Group Management Association Government Affairs Department. "CMMI Announces Payers in Comprehensive Primary Care Initiative." *MGMA Washington Connexion*, June 20, 2012, http://www.mgma.com/article.aspx?id=1371229 (accessed February 25, 2013).

Medical Group Management Association Government Affairs Department, "Final 2013 Medicare Physician Fee Schedule Lays Groundwork for Value-Based Payment Modifier." *Washington Link*, January 2013, pp. 20–22. http://www.mgma.com/workarea/downloadasset.aspx?id=1373088 (accessed January 24, 2013).

Midkiff, Herd, and Elizabeth Cordaro. "Developing Work RVUs for Production-Based Physician Compensation Programs." *hfm (Healthcare Financial Management)*, 66, no.6 (2012): 140–145.

Milburn, Jeffrey B. "Ease New Physicians into Productivity-Based Compensation Plans." *MGMA e-Source*, November. 9, 2010, http://mgma.com/article.aspx?id=39957 (accessed February 13, 2013).

Minich-Pourshadi, Karen. "Group Practice Innovators: Investing in Success." *HealthLeaders Media*, September 13, 2011, https://www.healthleadersmedia.com/page-5/MAG-270671/Group-Practice-Innovators-Investing-in-Success (accessed April 25, 2013).

Minich-Pourshadi, Karen. "Physician Compensation Incentives Shifting." *HealthLeaders Media*, October 28, 2011, http://www.healthleadersmedia.com/content/MAG-272014/Physician-Compensation-Incentives-Shifting.html (accessed February 17, 2013).

Minich-Pourshadi, Karen. "Return to the Employed Physician." *HealthLeaders Magazine*, 13, no.8 (2010): 29–30.

Molpus, Jim. "How Dean Clinic Redesigned Primary Care." *HealthLeaders Media*, April 22, 2013, http://www.healthleadersmedia.com/page-1/COM-291352/How-Dean-Clinic-Redesigned-Primary-Care (accessed April 25, 2013).

Mourar, Mary. *Experts Answer 95 New Practice Management* Questions. Englewood, CO: Medical Group Management Association, 2012.

Nash, Bruce, MD. "Rewarding Primary Care Practice Reform with Physician Payment Reform: A Medical Home's Experience." In *Guide to Physician Performance-Based Reimbursement: Payoffs from Incentives, Clinical Integration & Data Sharing*. Sea Girt, NJ: The Healthcare Intelligence Network, 2011, pp. 22–31.

NCQA Standards Workshop, Patient Centered Medical Home, PCMH 2011, http://www.ncqa.org/Portals/0/Programs/Recognition/RPtraining/PCMH%202011%20standards%201-3%20%20workshop_2.3.12.pdf (accessed April 5, 2013).

Pederson, Craig, and Theodore Praxel, MD. "Leveraging Marshfield Clinic's Practice Demonstration Experience in a "Value-Based" Environment." Presentation, MGMA 2011 Annual Conference, October 23–26, 2011.

Pierdon, Steven, and Brenda Eckrote. "Changing Compensation Plans Moving Beyond Last Year's, This Year's and Next Year's." *Physician Executive*, 30, no.1 (2004): 26–29.

Rainey, Jr., Willie F., MD, and Chrissy Van Erkelens, RN. "Genuine Quality and Service Incentives in a Physician P4P Program." *Group Practice Journal*, 59, no.8 (2010): 21, 24, 26–27.

Raskas, R.S., L.M. Latts, J.R. Hummel, D. Wenners, H. Levine, and S.R. Nussbaum. "Early Results Show WellPoint's Patient-Centered Medical Home Pilots Have Met Some Goals for Costs, Utilization, and Quality." *Health Affairs*, 31, no.9 (2012): 2002–2009.

Rodgers, Sally. "Restructuring Physician Compensation in an Academic Medical Setting." ACMPE Fellowship Paper, October 2009, https://www.mgma.com/workarea/mgma_downloadasset.aspx?id=34345 (accessed February 11, 2013).

Rousche, L. "Giving, and Getting, Back to Your Practice and Community." *Medical Economics*, 88, no.11 (2011): 53–54.

Samitt, Craig E., MD. "Rewarding Better Care at Lower Cost: Re-Designing MD Compensation in the World of Accountable Care." Health Industry Forum Presentation, October 22, 2012, http://healthforum.brandeis.edu/meetings/materials/2012-22-oct-CAPP1/2SamittHIF102212.pdf.pdf (accessed April 25, 2013).

Schmitt, John P., PhD, and Robert W. Keen, Esq. "Payer Contracting: Strategies to Boost Your Bottom Line While Preparing for Value-Based Contracts." MGMA webinar, October 11, 2012.

Souders, Jennifer L., FACMPE. "Establishing a Physician Compensation Plan." ACMPE Fellowship Paper, October 2011, http://www.mgma.com/workarea/mgma_downloadasset.aspx?id=1368495 (accessed January 8, 2013).

Stowell, Susan Reece, MBA, AVA, FACMPE. "Changing Incentives – Physician Compensation Under Health Reform." ACMPE Fellow Paper, 2011, http://www.mgma.com/workarea/downloadasset.aspx?id=1368310 (accessed January 18, 2013).

Weeks, William B., Stephen S. Rauh, Eric B. Wadsworth, and James N. Weinstein. "The Unintended Consequences of Bundled Payments." *Annals of Internal Medicine*, 158, no.1 (2013): 62–64.

Welle-Powell, Debbie, MPA. "Beyond Fee for Service – Moving to Episodes and Bundled Payments." MGMA webinar, June 2, 2011.

Westfall, Carol. "Group Culture: Medical Group Affiliation Levels and Effective Physician Recruitment." *NEJM CareerCenter Newsletter: Recruiting Physicians Today*, November-December 2003, www.nejmjobs.org/rpt/effective-physician-recruitment.aspx) (accessed February 1, 2013).

Whittenburg, Carl R., FACMPE. "Creating a Compensation Plan for an Academic Radiology Department." ACMPE Fellow Paper, October 2011, http://www.mgma.com/workarea/downloadasset.aspx?id=1368298 (accessed April 15, 2013).

"UnitedHealthcare Introduces New Cancer Care Payment Model." *Managed Care Outlook*, 23, no.24 (2010): 10–11.

Zuckerman, Alan M. *Health Care Strategic Planning*, 2nd edition. ACHE Management Series. Chicago, IL: Health Administration Press, 2005.

Index

Note: (ex.) indicates exhibit.

A

Academic faculty compensation, 171
  academic radiology department (case study), 187–188
  base salaries (rank- and tenure-based), 172–173
  and clinical activity, 171
  and competition with private practicing physicians, 171
  and complex organizational structure of academic medical centers, 172
  decline of guaranteed salaries, 173
  and decreased funding for teaching and research, 173
  funding sources, 171
  history of, 172–173
  MetroHealth Medical Center, Cleveland, OH (case study), 188–189
  plan implementation and review, 184–185
  and research grants, 171
  and state funding, 171
  traditionally lower than in private practice, 173
  triple mission (clinical, teaching, research), 171, 172
  University of Texas Southwestern Medical Center, Department of Surgery (case study), 186–187
  varying methodologies of, 172
Academic faculty compensation plan development, 173–174
  and administrative activities, 183
  and base salary plus incentives, 177–178
  and clinical activity and productivity compensation, 178
  compensation committee, 174–175
  compensation pool determination, 175–176, 183
  and faculty activities self-assessment form, 179–182, 181–182 (ex.)
  and faculty reporting form for hours and RVUs (example), 179–182, 180 (ex.)
  goals (sample), 174–175
  guiding principles (sample), 175
  incentive dollar amounts (points, RVUs), 184
  and incentive pool, 183, 183–184, 184 (ex.)
  and incentives, 176, 177–182
  and performance targets, 177–178
  salary alignment with marketplace (methods), 176–177
  salary system review, 176–178
  selection of committee members, 174

and teaching and research recognition, 178–182, 180 (ex.), 181–182 (ex.)
and teaching/research credits (points, RVUs), 179–182
and value-based reimbursement, 183
and wRVUs, 178
Academic medical centers (AMCs), 171, 172
and decreased funding for teaching and research, 173
and recruitment, 171
and retention, 171
Accountable care organizations (ACOs), 83–84, 137
Coastal Carolina Health Care, New Bern, NC (case study), 206–208
and Medicare Shared Savings Program (MSSP), 138–139
ProHealth Solutions, Waukesha, WI (case study), 208–210
and shared savings distributions, 140–141
and tax-exempt organizations, 139–140
Accreditation Association for Ambulatory Health Care, 82
Advocate Health System, Chicago, IL (integrated system), 211
Age Discrimination Act, 129
Agency for Healthcare Research and Quality (AHRQ), 80
Americans with Disabilities Act of 1990, 129–130
Anthem, Blue Precision (physician ranking), 40
Anti-Kickback Statute (federal; AKS), 130, 136–137
Employment Safe Harbor, 136–137
Personal Services and Management Contracts Safe Harbor, 137
safe harbors, 136–137
See also Stark law

B

Benchmarking, 34–35
and key indicators, 35
normalizing data, 36 (ex.)
as ongoing process, 36 (ex.)
and physician compensation and financial surveys, 35–37, 37 (ex.), 41–42
rules for, 35, 36 (ex.)
of service quality and patient satisfaction, 40–41
using applicable survey tables, 36 (ex.)
using median instead of mean, 36 (ex.)
Berwick, Don, 4
Billings Clinic, MT (productivity plus incentive system), 195–196
Blue Cross Blue Shield of Massachusetts, Alternative Quality Contract model, 87
Blue Cross Blue Shield of Minnesota, value-based initiative of, 77
Bonus payments, defined, 97
Bundled payments, 85–86

C

Call schedules and compensation
compensation types, 113, 114 (ex.)
dollar amount per call shift, 114
group practice call coverage, 113
hospital emergency call coverage, 113
reducing total compensation to reflect reduction in call, 114
RVU amount per call shift or hour, 114–115
Camino Medical Group, Calif. (multispecialty group), 212
Capital District Physicians' Health Plan medical home initiatives, 83
Capitation, 3–4, 14, 65
defined, 86
features of, 87
as risk-shifting inititative, 86–88
Care coordination initiatives, 13
CareFirst BlueCross BlueShield medical home initiatives, 83
Case rate payments, 14
Case rate reimbursement systems, 85
Centers for Medicare & Medicaid Services (CMS)

and accountable care organizations,
    83, 84
Bundled Payments for Care
    Improvement, 86
Comprehensive Primary Care
    Initiative, 81
Hierarchical Condition Category
    (HCC), 66
information resources, 216
Medicare value-based initiatives, 78–80
Physician Group Practice
    Demonstration project, 204
RBRVS lagging behind cost increases, 9
resource-based relative value scale
    (RBRVS), 9, 57–58, 59–60, 219–221
Risk Adjustment Factor (RAF), 66
Transitional Care Management codes,
    81
on value-based concept, 78
Cigna Collaborative Accountable Care
    initiative, 83, 204
Clinician and Group Consumer
    Assessment of Health Care Providers
    and Systems (CG-CAHPS) survey, 40,
    95, 199–200
Coastal Carolina Health Care, New Bern,
    NC (ACO incentives and shared
    savings distribution), 206–208
Compensation foundations
    (compensation in integrated
    systems)
  compensation per wRVU, 165
  and compensation regulations, 165
  guaranteed salary, 164
  incentives, 166–168
  productivity-based compensation, 16
Compensation foundations
    (compensation plan development),
    43
  and best practices in plan design,
    144–145
  and capital purchases, 44
  classified by complexity, 44, 45 (ex.)
  compensation pool, and accounting
    methodology, 44

compensation pool, and rolling
    averages of net operating profits,
    43, 44
compensation pool, calculating, 43–44
equal and productivity sharing, 53–54
equal share distribution, 47–49, 48 (ex.)
equal share plus incentive, 49–53
hybrid systems, 70–71, 71 (ex.)
with increasing complexity, 49–54
more complex, 54–71
productivity with expense allocation,
    66–70, 68 (ex.), 69 (ex.), 70 (ex.)
productivity-based, 54–66
and reserve funds, 44
salary plus incentive, 49–53
simple, 44–49
sizing up the alternatives, 43, 143–147
straight salary, 44–47
and tax issues, 44
and testing the draft plan, 145–146
transition or implementation plan,
    147
very complex, 71–72
See also Physician compensation plans
Compensation methodology goals and
    objectives, 22, 26 (ex.)
  aligning with organization's mission,
    vision, and culture, 22–24
  compensation plan guiding principles,
    25–26, 25 (ex.)
  compensation plan objectives, 24–26,
    25 (ex.)
  and physician input, 27–30, 27
    (ex.)–29 (ex.)
Compensation plan design in integrated
    systems
  Step 1. See Defining the problem or
    opportunity (compensation in
    integrated systems)
  Step 2. See Information needs
    (compensation in integrated
    systems)
  Step 3. See Data collection
    (compensation in integrated
    systems)

Step 4. *See* Data interpretation (compensation in integrated systems)

Step 5. *See* Compensation foundations (compensation in integrated systems)

Step 6. *See* Presenting the plan (compensation in integrated systems)

Step 7. *See* Determining outcome of the proposed plan (compensation in integrated systems)

Step 8. *See* Evaluating impact and outcome (compensation in integrated systems)

See also Integration of physicians and hospitals

Compensation plan development committee, 18

charge of, 19, 20 (ex.)

communication plan, 20–21

as distinct from governing body, 19

explaining reason for change, 21

governing body representation, 19

inclusion of outside consultant, 18, 19, 20 (ex.)

personnel included, 18–19

and physician buy-in vs. financial impacts, 21

status reports, 21

timeline, 19–20

Compensation plan development process, 17

Step 1. *See* Defining the problem or opportunity (compensation plan development)

Step 2. *See* Information needs (compensation plan development)

Step 3. *See* Data collection (compensation plan development)

Step 4. *See* Data interpretation (compensation plan development)

Step 5. *See* Compensation foundations (compensation plan development)

Step 6. *See* Presenting the plan (compensation plan development)

Step 7. *See* Determining outcome of the proposed plan (compensation plan development)

Step 8. *See* Evaluating impact and outcome (compensation plan development)

See also Compensation plan development committee

Contracts. *See* Physician employent agreements

CoxHealth, Springfield, MO

pay-for-performance plan, 196–199

physician performance report, 197–199, 198 (ex.)

D

Dartmouth-Hitchcock (integrated system with 20% incentive), 204–205

Data collection (compensation in integrated systems)

comparing apples to apples in benchmark reports, 163

physician surveys, 163

researching both private and integrated practices, 163

Data collection (compensation plan development), 31–32

on current practice situation, 32

financial, 32

on patient care, 32

payer analysis, 32–33

resources on compensation plans, 32

Data interpretation (compensation in integrated systems)

and hospital subsidization of physician compensation, 164

and physicians' trading lower compensation for reduced hassles, 164

Data interpretation (compensation plan development), 33

and benchmarking, 34–35, 40–41

comparison data analysis, 38–40, 39 (ex.)

and critical success factors in plans, 33–34

finalizing compensation plan goals and objectives, 41–42

and key indicators, 35

and MGMA DataDive modules, 36, 37 (ex.)

and physician compensation and financial surveys, 35–37, 37 (ex.)

DataDive modules, 36, 37 (ex.)

Physician Compensation and Production, 38

Dean Clinic, Madison, WI (value-based primary care), 199–200

Defining the problem or opportunity (compensation in integrated systems), 160

hospital priorities for physician employment and integration, 161

keys to negotiation success, 162–163

physician participation in plan design, 162

plan design committees, 161–163

plan goals and objectives, 160–161

and value-based incentive systems, 161

Defining the problem or opportunity (compensation plan development), 17

compensation methodology goals and objectives, 22–30, 25 (ex.), 26 (ex.)

compensation plan development committee, 18–21

determining plan's decision makers, 17–18

Designated health services (DHS) under Stark law, 131–132

Determining outcome of the proposed plan (compensation in integrated systems)

and need for physician input, 168

transition plan, 168

Determining outcome of the proposed plan (compensation plan development)

implementing plan, 150–151

modifications, based on physician input, 150

voting on plan, 150

Duluth Clinic, Duluth MN, (multispecialty group), 212

E

Equal and productivity sharing methodology, 53

advantages, 53

disadvantages, 54

Equal share distribution, 47

advantages, 48, 49

appropriate settings for, 48–49

calculating compensation pool, 47, 48 (ex.)

disadvantages, 48, 49–50

and performance expectations, 49

and physicians' direct expenses, 49

Equal share with incentive compensation formula (example), 50, 50 (ex.)

with value-based incentives, 71

Equity, internal and external, 24–25, 41

Evaluating impact and outcome (compensation in integrated systems)

monitoring measures analyzed in data collection and interpretation steps, 169

monitoring progress toward goals, 168–169

and physicians' sense of community, 169

post-implementation physician feedback, 169

Evaluating impact and outcome (compensation plan development), 151

auditing plan to ensure calculation accuracy, 151

comparing financial, coding, patient satisfaction data, etc., with pre-implementation data, 152

formal reviews at six months and one year, 151–152

monitoring need to rewrite or redevelop the compensation plan, 153–154

monitoring potential gaming of
system, 152–153
monitoring progress toward goals, 152
monitoring revenue, expenses, and
compensation distribution, 151
periodic status reports, 152
and transition from fee for service to
fee for quality, 153, 153 (ex.)
Evidence-informed Case Rate, 85

F
Fairness, 24–25, 41
Fee-for-service (FFS) model
problems with, 73–74
and shift to value-based compensation
incentives, 73
still dominant as value-based
incentives come into effect, 74

G
Geisinger Health System, Danville, PA
bundled payment program, 86
ProvenHealth Navigator (PCMH
program), 203
transition to patient-centered plan,
200–204
Global payments, 86
features of, 87
goal of, 87
and handling of out-of-network care,
88
key factors, 87–88
and member reconciliation (patient
attribution), 88
and scope of services or benefits
covered under contract, 88

H
Hawaii Medical Service Association,
shared savings program, 84
Health Care Incentives Improvement
Institute, Evidence-informed Case
Rate model, 85
Health Partners, Minneapolis, MN
(multispecialty group), 213

Healthcare expenditures
as percentage of gross domestic
product, 4 (ex.)
and value-based reimbursement, 4–5
HealthCare Partners Medical Group,
Calif. (multispecialty group), 212
Hierarchical Condition Category (HCC),
66
Humana, Provider Quality Rewards
program, 77
Hybrid compensation systems, 70–71,
71 (ex.)

I
Information needs (compensation in
integrated systems)
and federal and state regulations, 163
and organizational goals, mission, and
plans, 163
Information needs (compensation plan
development), 30
questions to identify, 30–31
Information resources
governmental, 216
MGMA-ACMPE, 215
on patient-centered medical homes,
216
on quality measures and guidelines,
217–218
Institute for Healthcare Improvement
(IHI), 4
Integration of physicians and hospitals,
155
achieving, 157
ACOs, 159
affiliation and integration models,
156–157, 175 (ex.)
and collections per RVU, 158
effects on physician income, 157–158
health system with control of
larger portion of physician
compensation, 159–160
and high level of integration, 159–160
hospitals' reasons for, 155–156
and incentives, 158–159

joint venture co-management, 158
and level of integration, 157 (ex.),
    158–160
and management service organizations
    (MSOs), 159
and moderate level of integration,
    158–159
payer encouragement of, 157
percentage of physician search
    assignments for hospital or health
    systems, 155, 156 (ex.)
physicians' reasons for, 156
and provider continuity, 157
service line management, 158
with set stipend, additional revenue
    options, or both, 158
See also Compensation plan design in
    integrated systems

J
Johns Hopkins, Guided Care program,
    81
The Joint Commission, 82

L
Late-career physicians, 113
Legal issues
    Age Discrimination Act, 129
    Americans with Disabilities Act of
        1990, 129–130
    Anti-Kickback Statute (AKS), 130,
        136–137
    avoiding discriminatory contract
        provisions, 129–130
    IRS rules for tax-exempt organizations,
        130
    IRS scrutinization of loans from
        practice to physicians,130–131
    Stark law, 130, 131–136
    taxation, 130
Lexington Clinic, KY (productivity plus
    incentive system), 196

M
Mayo Clinic, 47

Medicaid
    growth of, and changing payment
        systems, 11–12
    and Medicare as percentage of federal
        budget (2011), 4
    primary care payment parity rule,
        10–11
    See also Centers for Medicare &
        Medicaid Services
Medical homes. *See* Patient-centered
    medical homes
Medicare
    and accountable care organizations,
        83, 84
    Acute Care Episode program, 86
    and CG-CAHPS survey, 40, 95
    emphasis on primary and intensive
        care management, 10
    growth of, and changing payment
        systems, 11–12
    meaningful use requirement, 78–79
    and Medicaid as percentage of federal
        budget (2011), 4
    payment increases lagging behind
        Consumer Price Index, 9
    Physician Compare (ranking), 40
    Physician Quality Reporting System
        (PQRS), 12–13, 79, 96
    primary care payment parity rule,
        10–11
    sustainable growth rate (SGR) formula,
        9–10
    value-based initiatives, 78–80
    value-based payment modifier under
        Physician Fee Schedule, 79–80
    value-based reimbursement modifier,
        12–13
    See also Centers for Medicare &
        Medicaid Services; Stark law
Medicare Payment Advisory
    Commission, 10
Medicare Shared Savings Program
    (MSSP), 137
    and shared savings distributions to
        ACO participants, 140–141

and tax-exempt organizations, 139–140
waivers, 138–139
MetroHealth Medical Center, Cleveland, OH, 188–189
MGMA DataDive modules, 36, 37 (ex.)
Physician Compensation and Production, 38
MGMA Medical Directorship and On-Call Compensation Survey, 114
MGMA Performance and Practices of Successful Medical Groups, 36
MGMA Physician Compensation and Production Survey, 110
MGMA Physician Placement and Starting Salary Survey, 47
MGMA-ACMPE information resources, 215
Mid-career physicians, 112–113
Mission statements, 22–24, 25 (ex.)
Mount Auburn Hospital, Cambridge, MA (integrated system), 211

N
National Committee for Quality Assurance (NCQA)
Healthcare Effectiveness Data and Information Set (HEDIS), 77, 87
medical home accreditation, 82
National Quality Forum (NQF), "Community Tool to Align Measurement," 92
New physicians
and building of patient panel and referral base, 108–109
determining salary level, 109–110, 110 (ex.), 111
experienced and newly recruited, 111
and guaranteed salary, 109
need for initial support from practice, 108–109
physician couple sharing one full-time equivalent position, 111
practice ownership and buy-in issues, 111–112

recruitment packages (signing bonus, student loan help, etc.), 110
transition to productivity-based plan, 109, 110–112
of two-physician families, 111
Nonphysician providers (NPPs), 8–9
and physician compensation for supervision of, 116–117, 117 (ex.)
Nurse anesthetists, 8
Nurse practitioners, 8

O
Obamacare. *See* Patient Protection and Affordable Care Act of 2010

P
Panel size. *See* Patient panel size
Part-time physicians, 115
and expense allocation, 116
job sharing, 111, 116
methods used to accommodate, 115–116, 115 (ex.)
Partners HealthCare, Boston, MA (multispecialty group), 213
Patient centeredness, defined, 80–81
Patient encounters as productivity measure
advantages, 64
ambulatory, 63–64
appropriate settings for use of, 64
defined, 63
disadvantages, 64
hospital, 63
using total or ambulatory, 64
Patient panel size as productivity measure
appropriate settings for use of, 65
and capitation, 65
and cost and/or utilization management, 65
defined, 64
and payment based on per beneficiary (member) per month (PMPM), 65
and severity of illness, 65–66

Patient Protection and Affordable Care Act of 2010 (PPACA), 4, 10, 11
and accountable care organizations, 137–138
Patient-centered medical homes (PMCHs), 13
certification organizations, 81–82
defined, 81
Geisinger Health System program, 203
information resources, 216
per member per month (PMPM) reimbursement, 82
reimbursement methods for, 82–83, 82 (ex.)
Pay-for-performance. *See* Value-based reimbursement
Payer incentive plans
history of, 74–75
introduction of multiple plans in largely FFS environment, 74
lack of transparency in, 74–75
from Medicare and others, 73
shift toward value, not volume, 73–74
Per beneficiary (member) per month (PMPM), 65, 82–83, 86
Physician assistants, 8
Physician compensation plan design
best practices, 144–145
testing the draft plan, 145–146
and transition or implementation plan, 147
Physician compensation plans, 1
and accountable care organizations (ACOs), 13
for administrative duties, 119–120
and behavioral incentives or penalties, 123
and call schedules, 113–115, 114 (ex.)
capitated managed care, 3–4
and care coordination initiatives, 13
change in median compensation 2008–2012, 11, 11 (ex.)
and changing demand for physician services, 10–11

and citizenship activities, 121
and committee activities, 121
and cost increases exceeding reimbursement rate increases, 9–10
development of, 2
external challenges, 9–15
and formation of larger practices, 8
and generational or gender issues, 8
historical perspective, 2–4
importance of, 5
and incentives, 3
and integration/alignment with hospitals, 14–15
and internal challenges, 8–9
and large group practices, 118–119
and leadership incentives, 120
for managing partners, 119–120
for medical directors, 119–120, 120 (ex.)
and medical homes, 13
and merging practices into a larger group, 118–119
and new physicians, 108–112
and new reimbursement initiatives, 11–14
and nonphysician providers, 8–9
objectives, 1
and part-time physicians, 111, 115–116
and physician behavior, 1–3
and physician self-esteem, 1
and physician shortages, 11
and physicians' career stages, 108–113
and practice culture, 9
and practice leadership and administration, 9
productivity-based (fee-for-service), 3, 4
and revenues from activities outside of the practice, 121–122
and rising costs, 8
and risk-shifting reimbursement systems, 13–14
and shared savings programs, 13
sharing of revenue in groups, 2

special issues, 107–108

special issues, compensation pool for, 124

specialist income in group practices, 118

and subjective measures (peer rating, employee satisfaction, etc.), 123

and supervision of nonphysician providers (NPPs), 116–117, 117 (ex.)

traditional ("keep what you treat"), 2

value-based reimbursement (pay-for-performance), 4–5, 12–13

and volunteer community service, 122

when to devise new plan, 6–7

when to review and modify, 5–7, 6 (ex.)

See also Compensation foundations; Compensation methodology goals and objectives; Compensation plan design in integrated systems; Compensation plan development committee; Compensation plan development process; Productivity-based compensation; Value-based incentives and physician compensation

Physician compensation system questionnaire, 27, 27 (ex.)–29 (ex.)

Physician employment agreements

addenda re compensation provisions, 128

alignment with group's goals and mission, 126

avoiding discriminatory language, 129–130

avoiding legalese and ambiguity, 127

boilerplate provisions, 129

bonuses and special payments treated as loans, 128

corporation's rights, duties, and obligations, 129

forming, 125–126

keeping signed copy in accessible but confidential place, 126

length of time of, 129

negotiation by board or executive, 126

no-compete covenants, 128

obligations of group and physician upon termination, 128

physician's duties, 129

termination provisions, 127–128, 129

terms of, 126–127

typical provisions, 128–129

Physician Quality Reporting System (Medicare), 79, 96

Physicians' career stages and compensation

late-career physicians, 113

mid-career physicians, 112–113

new physicians, 108–112

PMCHs. *See* Patient-centered medical homes

PMPM. *See* Per beneficiary (member) per month

PPACA. *See* Patient Protection and Affordable Care Act of 2010

Practice culture, 9, 22–24

Practice mission statement, 22–24, 25 (ex.)

Practice vision statement, 22–24

Presenting the plan (compensation in integrated systems), 168

Presenting the plan (compensation plan development), 147–149

presenting physician-specific numbers (reports and scorecards), 149

Primary care initiatives, 80

care management and coordination, 81

medical homes, 81–83

and patient centeredness, 80–81

Primary care physicians (PCPs), need for and changing compensation of, 11, 11 (ex.)

PriMed (multispecialty group), 212

Private payer initiatives, 76–77

examples, 77–78

key criteria, 77

new reimbursement models, 78

Private payers, and RVUs and RBRVS system, 221

Productivity with expense allocation, 66
  direct allocation, 67
  and direct expenses, 66
  equal share allocation, 67, 68 (ex.)
  expense allocation options, 67–70
  and fixed expenses, 66
  and indirect expenses, 66–67
  mix of equal and direct allocation, 69
  plus value-based incentives, 71
  productivity-based allocation, 68,
    69 (ex.)
  RVU expense allocation, 69–70, 70 (ex.)
  and variable expenses, 66
Productivity-based compensation, 54
  advantages, 55
  appropriate settings for, 55–56
  basic compensation formula, 54
  and charges (professional gross
    charges), 56
  and collections (gross revenue), 57
  disadvantages, 55
  and patient encounters, 63–64
  and patient panel size, 64–66
  productivity measures, 56–66
  and work relative value units (wRVUs),
    57–63, 60 (ex.), 61 (ex.), 62 (ex.),
    63 (ex.)
  See also Value-based incentives and
    physician compensation
ProHealth Solutions, Waukesha, WI,
  208–210
Prometheus Payment model, 85

R
RAF. See Risk Adjustment Factor
RBRVS. See Resource-based relative value
  scale
Reimbursement models
  accountable care organizations
    (ACOs), 83–84
  and fee-for-service (FFS) system, 73–74
  four main models of new systems, 75
  Medicare value-based initiatives, 78–80
  patient-centered and primary care
    initiatives, 80–83

private payer initiatives, 76–78
  risk-shifting initiatives, 84–88
  shared savings programs, 83–84
  and value-based compensation
    incentives, 73–74
  value-based reimbursement, 75–76
Relative value units (RVUs), 58
  advantages, 58–59
  calculation components, 58
  in compensation per call shift or hour
    on call, 114–115
  disadvantages, 59
  explanation of, 219–221
  Medicare conversion factor, 58
Resource-based relative value scale
  (RBRVS), 9, 57–58, 59–60
  explanation of, 219–221
Risk Adjustment Factor (RAF), 66
Risk-shifting initiatives, 84–85
  bundled payments, 85–86
  capitation and global payments, 86–88
  case rate reimbursement systems, 85
  and physician compensation, 88
Risk-shifting reimbursement systems,
  13–14

S
Salary plus incentive, 49–50
  advantages, 51
  appropriate settings for, 51
  calculating compensation pool, 50–51
  compensation formula (example), 50,
    50 (ex.)
  disadvantages, 51
  and disadvantages of straight salary,
    49–50
  incentive selection, 51–52
  objective incentive measures, 51–52
  and patient satisfaction measurement,
    52
  percentage of compensation for
    incentives, 52–53
  subjective incentive measures, 52
  and team goals, 53
  with value-based incentives, 71

Shared savings programs, 13, 83–84
    Coastal Carolina Health Care, New
        Bern, NC (case study), 206–208
Southeast Permanente Medical Group,
    Atlanta, GA, 205
Stark law, 130, 133
    definition of group practice, 132–133
    and designated health services (DHS),
        131–132
    entity, defined, 132
    exceptions to, 132
    key provision of, 131
    and Medicare revenue, 131
    and "overall profits," 135
    and profit distributions to
        shareholders, 112, 121
    and providing DHS services within a
        practice, 132
    rules for productivity bonuses, 133–134
    rules for profit sharing, 135–136
    safe harbors re productivity bonuses,
        133–134
    safe harbors re profit sharing, 135
    and services "incident to" physician's
        services, 134
    and subsets of group practice, 135
Straight salary, 44
    advantages, 45, 47
    appropriate settings for, 46
    calculating compensation pool, 46
    disadvantages, 45, 47, 49–50
    within fair market value, but
        affordable, 46
    lack of productivity incentives, 47
    for new physicians, 47

T

Taxation issues, 130
    IRS rules for tax-exempt organizations,
        130
    IRS scrutinization of loans from
        practice to physicians,130–131
Texas, University of, Southwestern
    Medical Center, Department of
    Surgery, 186–187
Triple Aim, 4–5

U

UnitedHealthcare
    bundled payment program, 86
    UnitedHealth Premium (physician
        ranking), 40
    value-based initiative (Illinois), 77
URAC, 82

V

Value-based factors (case studies)
    ACO incentives and shared savings
        distribution, 206–210
    Advocate Health System, Chicago, IL
        (integrated system), 211
    base salary with tiered RVU incentive,
        194–195
    Billings Clinic, MT (productivity plus
        incentive), 195–196
    Camino Medical Group, Calif.
        (multispecialty group), 212
    Coastal Carolina Health Care, New
        Bern, NC (incentives and shared
        savings distribution), 206–208
    complex methodology with value-
        based incentives, 196–205
    CoxHealth, Springfield, MO (pay-for-
        performance plan), 196–199,
        198 (ex.)
    Dartmouth-Hitchcock (integrated
        system with incentive), 204–205
    Dean Clinic, Madison, WI (value-
        based primary care), 199–200
    Duluth Clinic, Duluth MN,
        (multispecialty group), 212
    equal share distribution, 191–192
    family practice group (salary +
        incentive), 193–194
    Geisinger Health System, Danville,
        PA (transition to patient-centered
        plan), 200–204
    Health Partners, Minneapolis, MN,
        (multispecialty group), 213
    HealthCare Partners Medical Group,
        Calif. (multispecialty group), 212
    integrated system models, 211–213

integrated system with 20% incentive, 204–205

large multispecialty practices, 212–213

Lexington Clinic, KY (productivity plus incentive), 196

more complex methodologies, 195–205

Mount Auburn Hospital, Cambridge, MA (integrated system), 211

Partners HealthCare, Boston, MA (multispecialty group), 213

and primary care, 199–200

PriMed (multispecialty group), 212

productivity plus incentive, 195–196

ProHealth Solutions, Waukesha, WI (incentives and shared savings distribution), 208–210

quality-adjusted RVU method, 205

salary plus incentive, 192–195

simple compensation methodologies, 191–195

Southeast Permanente Medical Group, Atlanta, GA (quality-adjusted RVU method), 205

three-physician practice (salary + incentive), 192–193

transition to patient-centered plan, 200–204

Value-based incentives, 71–72

and cost and utilization control incentives, 103–104

distributed separately from regular compensation, 150–151

implementation of the plan, 104

and patients' health outcomes or health status measures, 103

and subjectivity of patient satisfaction, 102–103

and unforeseen consequences, 102–104

Value-based incentives and physician compensation, 88–90

bonus or incentive payments, 97

and CG-CAHPS survey, 95

deciding if reward is based on target achievement, improvement, or maintenance, 100–101

determining individual, team, or organizational measures and incentives, 96–97

determining weighting of measures, 99–100, 99 (ex.), 100 (ex.)

differences between FFS and value-based reimbursement, 89, 89 (ex.)

establishing size and source of incentive pool, 97–99

identifying data sources, 95–96

identifying incentive payment mechanism, 101–102

incentive compensation options, 99, 100 (ex.)

incentive plan development, steps in, 90–102

in mixed FFS and value-based environment, 89–90

patient satisfaction goals, 95–96

and performance reports or scorecards, 96

and Physician Quality Reporting System, 96

selecting value-based metrics, 91–96

value-based metrics (examples), 92, 93 (ex.)

and wRVUs, 99–100

See also Productivity-based compensation

Value-based reimbursement, 4–5

and benchmarking, 76

defined, 75–76

FFS or capitation combined with performance incentives, 76

modifier, 12–13

and performance targets, 76

Vision statements, 22–24

W

WellPoint medical home initiatives, 82–83

Work relative value units (wRVUs), 57

in academic faculty compensation, 178

advantages, 58–59

base salary plus tiered sRVU values,
61–63, 62 (ex.)
calculation components, 58
compensation-to-wRVU ratios and use
of percentiles, 62, 63 (ex.)
in determining incentive payments to
physicians, 99–100
disadvantages, 59, 63
ensuring accurated RVU calculations,
59, 60 (ex.)
and expertise in Medicare RBRVS
system, 59

individual wRVUs as percentage of
group wRVUs, 61, 61 (ex.)
individual wRVUs times compensation
ratio, 61, 61 (ex.), 62, 223–225,
223 (ex.), 224 (ex.), 225 (ex.)
and Medicare conversion factor, 58
modifying values to reflect practice's
priorities, 60–61
and RBRVS system adjustments, 59–60

About the Authors

Jeffrey B. Milburn, MBA, CMPE

Formerly the senior vice president and interim chief executive officer of a 90-physician multispecialty group, Jeffrey B. Milburn, CMPE, has more than 25 years of healthcare management experience. He has served as a chief financial officer and held responsibility for his organization's payer contracting and management. Before entering the healthcare field, he worked for 10 years in the commercial banking and finance field.

Jeff has presented programs and workshops on a variety of healthcare topics and provided editorial assistance on a number of publications related to healthcare financial management. His areas of expertise include physician compensation, financial benchmarking, financial management, and payer contracting. He is the recipient of the 2007 ACMPE Edward B. Stevens Article of the Year Award for his article, "Mining for Gold: Extract Revenue from Unprocessed Claim Denials."

Mary Mourar, MLS

Mary Mourar is a healthcare information professional, freelance writer, and developmental editor. While working for MGMA for more than 11 years as a librarian and information specialist in the MGMA Knowledge Center, Mary assisted MGMA members and staff with a plethora of medical practice management questions, addressing current trends and issues across the healthcare industry. She has written and edited several books for MGMA. Mary received a master's degree in library science from the University of California at Los Angeles and a bachelor of arts degree from Colorado College.